GESTAT

DIABETES

Deborah Hughes

AİMS

Published by AIMS
www.aims.org.uk
publications@aims.org.uk
Tel: 0300 365 0663

© AIMS 2017
Association for Improvements in the Maternity Services
Registered Charity number 1157845
ISBN: 978-1-874413-39-4

Artwork by Jennifer Williams

A note on the cover illustration: expectant mothers share a great deal with each other, but nurture their own hopes, expectations and horizons.

Printed in the Czech Republic by Printo

About AIMS

The Association for Improvements in the Maternity Services (AIMS) has been at the forefront of the childbirth movement since 1960. Run entirely by unpaid volunteers, it became a Registered Charity in 2014.

AIMS' day-to-day work includes providing independent support and information about maternity choices and raising awareness of current research on childbirth and related issues. AIMS actively supports parents and healthcare professionals who recognise that, for the majority of women, birth is normal rather than a medical event. AIMS campaigns tirelessly on many issues covered by the Human Rights legislation.

Author's acknowledgements

With thanks to Mary White, my long-time walking companion, for reading this through when it wasn't really readable; to Professor Helen Murphy of the University of East Anglia, whose knowledge of and passion for diabetes and pregnancy is a national resource; to Professor David Simmons of the University of Western Sydney, who gave me a job when I needed one and got me interested in GDM; to Debbie Chippington Derrick of AIMS and the production team, Shane Ridley, Gina Lowdon and Alison Melvin, who made it all happen; to Angie Barrett for reading it through with her midwife's eyes; to Jennifer Williams for livening it up with her lovely drawings; to the women who took part in the DALI Study at Cambridge University Hospitals Trust and in whose journeys I shared; and, last but not least, to the women who have shared their stories in this book.

Deborah Hughes

CONTENTS

About AIMS   iii

Author's acknowledgements   iv

Foreword   1

Introduction   3

The increasing diagnosis of gestational diabetes and the choices
and decisions around it   3

Chapter 1: What is GDM?   7

What are the problems associated with GDM, and can it be
prevented?   7

Insulin and 'Insulin-resistance': the key to GDM   7

What is 'normal' blood glucose in pregnancy?   10

BMI, Ethnicity and GDM   10

Hyperglycaemia of pregnancy and birth outcomes   13

Preventing GDM when you are already pregnant – the research
so far   17

Lifestyle changes (diet and exercise)   *18*

Vitamin D supplementation   *20*

Drugs   *22*

Alternatives   *22*

Chapter 2:
Having the test for GDM - is it for you?   **24**

Blood tests for gestational diabetes and diabetes   24

Being offered a test for gestational diabetes in pregnancy   27

What tests are offered?   29

Deciding whether to have a blood test for GDM   29

Having the test for GDM: going for an OGTT   32

Women's Experiences   *35*

Chapter 3:
Making sense of the test results   **41**

Getting the results   41

Diabetes Mellitus: being diagnosed with diabetes for the first time
when you are pregnant   41

Being diagnosed with gestational diabetes mellitus (GDM) during
pregnancy   43

Working out if you have GDM – it all depends where you are!
Sort of...   47

Odds Ratios (for readers who enjoy statistics)   *50*

Chapter 4:
Being diagnosed with GDM – what next?   **51**

Care and Treatment for GDM:
the first appointment   51

Care and Treatment for GDM:
the second appointment   58

Ongoing care and interventions, including treatment with
metformin or insulin   59

    The BRAIN approach to health decisions   *63*

Medication for GDM   65

    Metformin   *65*

    Insulin   *67*

    Glibenclamide   *70*

If you are admitted to hospital during pregnancy   70

Induction of labour   71

Blood glucose monitoring and control during labour   77

    The BRAIN approach to considering induction of labour: *77*

    Women's Experiences   *78*

Chapter 5:
Postnatal Care - the first few days   **89**

    Looking after yourself   89

    Feeding your baby and managing newborn hypoglycaemia   89

    If your baby needs special care on a neonatal unit   97

    Womens' Experiences   *99*

Chapter 6:
Preventing Diabetes after GDM   **102**

    What should I do after I have had GDM?
    What are the longer-term implications of GDM?   102

Testing plasma glucose levels after having GDM and what the
results mean   102

Preventing type 2 diabetes after having GDM: breastfeeding,
lifestyle change, drug therapy   104

  Breastfeeding   105

  Lifestyle change   106

  Drugs   109

  Women's Experiences   110

E-resources and Social Media   **111**

Glossary   **117**

References   **124**

About the Author   **131**

About the Illustrator   **131**

Foreword

AIMS receives a great many requests for information from women who have been diagnosed with Gestational Diabetes (GD) or are faced with the decision about whether to be tested for it. We know from the AIMS helpline and social media that questions about GD are a concern for a significant number of women and that there is pressure for women to submit to routine care as set out in hospital guidelines. We hear frequently from women that they do not have the information they need to make decisions.

We hope this book will help you to understand the issues and the research on GD, as well as the tests, treatments and options you have before you decide on what you need and want from your health care professionals. You will be able to read about other women's experiences too, to show you how varied these, and the decisions they take, can be.

We are very grateful to Deborah Hughes, an experienced and respected midwife, for taking on this very complex subject. She carefully takes the reader through what is known about the risks, and what may be of help in terms of lifestyle changes and treatments. We believe this book will make it much easier for women to understand what is happening to them, what the risks and benefits may be of being tested and of the treatments available.

Deborah shows how women can make informed decisions about whether they wish to accept or decline testing or treatment, but also whether to accept interventions, for example, induction of labour which is often offered to women who are diagnosed with GD.

We are delighted that Jennifer Williams agreed to work with Deborah to provide the helpful infographics and insightful, often funny, illustrations which bring the book to life.

You may feel a bit shocked at being diagnosed with or even just told you might have GD, especially in your first pregnancy when you have so many other things to think about. By using this book, you will be able to make your own assessment of the risks and benefits for you for all the different options available. At AIMS we know that one size *doesn't* fit all.

The AIMS Committee

Introduction

The increasing diagnosis of gestational diabetes and the choices and decisions around it

This book is for anyone who has been diagnosed with **gestational diabetes mellitus (GDM)**[1] or for anyone who is trying to decide whether or not to accept testing for GDM. Testing for GDM is now a routine part of antenatal care, and more women than ever before are being diagnosed with GDM. The issues associated with testing and diagnosis are thoroughly explored in this book.

The rise in the number of women diagnosed with GDM isn't just a UK phenomenon: rates of GDM are increasing across the world, closely linked to changes in lifestyle and food availability that have led to higher **body mass indexes (BMIs)** and particularly increases in body fat. As we get fatter, we are more likely to develop diabetes and this includes diabetes associated with pregnancy. In addition to this, testing for GDM has also increased. It is hard to know how much of the increase in GDM is down to a rise in actual incidence and how much is down to more women being tested; it is likely to be a mixture of the two.

Furthermore, different diagnostic criteria are used. How test results are evaluated in one hospital or one country to diagnose GDM may differ from those in your local hospital or in your country. This means that the thresholds at which women are given a diagnosis of GDM differ from place-to-place (I shall discuss this in Chapter 3).

---

1 Words or terms in **bold** in the text can be found in the Glossary on page 117.

At the time of writing (2017), in the UK around 1 in 18 pregnant women (roughly 40,000) are diagnosed with GDM each year and the number is rising annually. In Australia, the rate is very similar. For women with a BMI greater than 30, the rate rises to 1 in 4.

Some ethnic groups are more likely to develop GDM and in Bradford, UK, where a large proportion of the population is of South Asian descent, the rate is almost 1 in 5 (Farrar *et al.*, 2015). I talk more about ethnicity and GDM in Chapter 1.

So, if you are reading this having been diagnosed with GDM, you are NOT alone. You are very likely to know or find someone else who has been diagnosed with GDM at work, at college, in your local playgroup or antenatal class, or through your social media networks, and you will be able to discuss thoughts and experiences with them.

GDM is a complex issue and, as we shall explore in this book, it is very much bound up with the concept of **'risk'**. Whilst I shall attempt to quantify some of the risks associated with GDM, risk is something we all understand differently, and interpret according to our personal views. For example, nothing would induce me to accept the risks associated with bungee-jumping or snake-keeping, but other people, even close friends, interpret the risks about such things, and make choices about them, very differently. On the other hand, I may accept risks that they think are foolhardy, such as swimming across a river or not going for mammograms. It isn't simply about knowing what the risk of something is (e.g. 1 in 4, 1 in 400, 1 in 40,000), but also about what value we attach to the activity and the risk associated with it on a personal level. This is a highly individual process, related to our beliefs, past experiences, aspirations and values.

In any given situation requiring a decision or choice to be made, what may be right for me will not be right for you, and neither of our decisions or choices may be right for the next person. In health care, there is a tendency to take what an expert advises as right or correct and the only possible course to follow. However, a health care professional's advice may be biased, it may be out-of-date, it may be their personal opinion or what makes them feel most comfortable; it may be what they would do in your situation or what they think you want to do, or it may be inspired by a great article they read in a medical journal over breakfast! You need to weigh up what you have been told and to ask questions on any area that you are unclear about.

We all feel happier with some health professionals than we do with others, and we know that some of those we see are brilliant in their field but others are less so. Our health care decisions are taken against this backdrop of personal experience, our situation, values and beliefs, and what we know and how we feel about those caring for us. To make life more complicated, there is always a large area of uncertainty around most areas of health care – much is unknown, all the factors that affect outcomes are unclear, there is a mixed bag of research evidence on many topics, there is more than one way of approaching most problems, and there are advantages and disadvantages in various proportions to nearly every treatment or intervention; thus a personal decision is essential.

This book will highlight the areas where decisions and choices arise and what you may want to consider when making your choices, with some suggestions on reaching a decision. It will become obvious to you that, whilst there is quite a lot of research on GDM, there is much that remains unknown, unclear or inconclusive, and findings from one study may not entirely agree with or confirm those from another. I have tried to provide the most up-to-date and broadly relevant studies and to identify where some agreement exists as to what is helpful for women and babies. But even so, there is always room for personal decision-making – remember it is YOUR body, YOUR baby, YOUR life. Research is based on large groups of women, a 'population' of however many women took part in a study. It is always difficult to apply findings from one such 'population' to you as an individual, but only YOU, with the help of friends, family and health professionals if you want it, decide to what extent they apply to YOU.

Some GDM pregnancy stories from AIMS Facebook readers are included at the end of some chapters, and these may help you on your own journey.

You may find another AIMS publication helpful when considering some of the main decisions around maternity care. *Am I Allowed?* by Beverley Lawrence Beech helps you explore your rights and the issues of autonomy, consent and the law when pregnant and giving birth, and looks at the main areas of choice in maternity care.

Finally, gestational diabetes is a complex topic and discussion of it is not easy. I have done my best to make the subject understandable, whilst not over-simplifying it. I hope that I have been able to achieve this and please do remember that the volunteers from AIMS are always here to help you with decisions, as these evolve and change, without any pressure.

Chapter 1: What is GDM?

What are the problems associated with GDM, and can it be prevented?

Insulin and 'Insulin-resistance': the key to GDM

Pregnancy is a time of considerable hormonal change, as you are likely to be well aware! One of the effects of these hormonal changes is that your body cells become more 'resistant' to insulin. **Insulin** is a hormone made by the pancreas and it plays a very important part in helping cells use the energy we take into our bodies when we eat **carbohydrates**. Carbohydrates exist in many foods, but make up a high proportion of foods such as starchy vegetables (potatoes, squash etc.) and grains (rice, bread, pasta etc.). The various sugars (glucose, lactose, fructose etc.) are solely carbohydrate.

Our body converts carbohydrates to the **glucose** that our cells and our unborn baby's cells use for energy; glucose is the fuel that our bodies run on. Insulin is essential to enable our body cells to take in and use glucose from the blood stream; without insulin the cells cannot function. **Insulin resistance** means that insulin does not have the same level of effect on the body's cells. When you are pregnant the cells are naturally less efficient at taking in glucose; in other words, the cells 'resist' insulin to some degree, and this is a normal part of pregnancy. The insulin resistance of pregnancy, caused by pregnancy hormones, is a natural phenomenon and probably plays a role in ensuring fetal well-being and growth by enabling glucose to remain in the mother's blood for longer periods. In this way, the fetus always has access to sufficient glucose for its growth needs. To compensate for this insulin resistance, the **pancreas** produces even more insulin to ensure that overall levels of blood glucose are maintained within normal limits whilst also allowing the baby to get what it needs from the greater availability of glucose. This pregnancy-related 'super-production' of insulin is called **hyperinsulinaemia**.

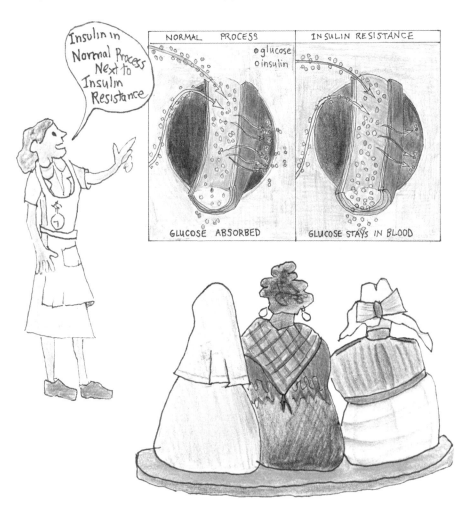

So, increased insulin resistance, some degree of more readily-available blood glucose for the baby, and an increase in insulin production to keep this under control, are normal in pregnancy and differ slightly between individual women because physiological needs vary to some extent.

However, these adaptive processes are not fully understood. The uncertainty has led to some people dismissing GDM as 'a label in search of a disease', believing both screening and diagnosis to be a misunderstanding of the physiology of pregnancy. At the other end of the spectrum is universal screening for GDM and treating all women diagnosed with GDM as high risk. The picture is more complicated than either position and this is why making decisions and choices has to be personal and individual and what this book hopes to help you to do.

For most women, the normal hyperinsulinaemia of pregnancy is able to balance the pregnant body's insulin-resistance, the need for continuous glucose availability for baby, and prevents the build-up of excess glucose in the mother's blood. But some pregnant women do not produce enough insulin to overcome their insulin-resistance, and their blood glucose levels rise. When this happens, they develop a diabetes-like condition known as gestational diabetes or GDM. This tends to occur later in pregnancy and that is why tests for GDM are mainly done around the 24th to 28th week. (For more on the timing of tests for GDM, see Chapter 2.) As the mother's higher glucose levels cross the placenta, they lead to increased insulin production or hyperinsulaemia in the fetus, as the baby's body tries to counteract the extra glucose. I will talk more about this later, especially in Chapters 4 and 5.

What is 'normal' blood glucose in pregnancy?

Quite a lot of effort has gone into establishing the normal blood glucose level for pregnancy, and it is concluded to be **between 4 and 6mmol/L**[2], although it is not unusual for it to drop to 3.5mmol/L in early pregnancy (Hernandez et al., 2011). Hernandez and colleagues examined data from 12 studies that asked women between 24 and 40 weeks of pregnancy to monitor their blood glucose levels throughout the day over a period of time. The women had normal pregnancies and were not overweight. Findings from all the studies were remarkably consistent and, when all the blood glucose levels were charted, they clearly demonstrated a very similar pattern and very narrow range of glucose levels. The average blood glucose in the 255 women who took part in the studies was:

Fasting: 3.9mmol/L
1 hour after a meal: 6.1mmol/L
2 hours after a meal: 5.5mmol/L
Mean blood glucose (over 24 hours): 4.9mmol/L

Using a calculation called standard deviation, these results have been used to set some suggested targets for women to aim for when they have GDM (these will be discussed in Chapter 4).

BMI, Ethnicity and GDM

It is not just pregnancy hormones that cause insulin resistance; body-fat is also insulin resistant and sometimes results in higher blood glucose levels. This is why **type 2 diabetes** is more common in people who

---

2 mmol/L means millimoles per litre of blood and is how blood glucose levels are usually measured in the UK.

are classified as overweight. Pregnant women who are overweight (a pre-pregnancy **Body Mass Index** or **BMI** above 25) are more likely to have a greater degree of insulin-resistance (a double-whammy of insulin-resistance so to speak) than those with lower BMIs. This is why it is more likely that you will be diagnosed with 'gestational diabetes' if your BMI is high.

So to give you an idea of this additional likelihood of having GDM if you are a bigger woman, here is an approximate guide. If you are 'overweight' (BMI of 25 to 30) you are twice as likely to be diagnosed with GDM as someone with a BMI of 20 to 25. If you are 'obese' (BMI of 30 to 35), you are 4 times as likely to be diagnosed with GDM (1 in 4 women will develop GDM at this BMI), and if you are 'severely obese' (BMI above 35), you are 8 times as likely to develop GDM as someone with a 'healthy' BMI (1 in 2 women will develop GDM at this BMI) (Chu et al., 2007). [I use these BMI classifications here for convenience whilst recognising there are problems with this terminology.]

However, you may be diagnosed with gestational diabetes even if your BMI is low, especially if you come from a black or Asian minority ethnic group. This is partly due to a greater genetic tendency to diabetes in certain ethnic groups, including those from the Asian subcontinent (Pakistan, India, Sri Lanka and Bangladesh), but also to the fact that some ethnic groups (like those just mentioned) tend to have more body fat for any given BMI.

If you are from a black African or Caribbean background, you are 2 to 3 times more likely to develop GDM than a woman from a white British background with the same BMI. If you are from a south Asian background (Pakistani, Bangladeshi, Indian) then you are about 3 to 4 times more likely to develop GDM than a woman from a white British background at the same BMI (Yuen & Wong, 2015; Farrar *et al.*, 2015). Precise percentages are hard to come by, but around 5% of women from white British backgrounds develop GDM, around 11% of women from black African or Afro-Caribbean backgrounds and about 15% of women from a south Asian background. Similar differences in rates exist amongst ethnic groups in both North America and Australia/ New Zealand due to various combinations of genetics and lifestyles that are poorly understood.

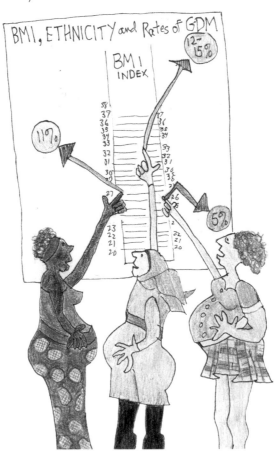

This is not to say that you cannot be from, say, an Indian background, have a BMI of 35 and not have GDM. Even then, you stand a reasonable chance (probably almost 1 in 2) of not having it, but knowing that you are at an increased risk may help you decide what you want to do when you are faced with choices around GDM screening.

Hyperglycaemia of pregnancy and birth outcomes

Abnormally high levels of of glucose in the blood is known as **hyperglycaemia**. Hyperglycaemia of pregnancy occurs when the degree of insulin being produced in a woman's body is not enough to overcome her insulin resistance and keep her blood glucose within normal levels, as described at the beginning of this chapter.

A few women are diagnosed with diabetes (either **type 1 diabetes** or **type 2 diabetes**) for the first time when they are pregnant. Either their insulin levels are very low and their antibody results show that they have type 1 diabetes, an auto-immune disease causing the pancreas to stop producing insulin, or their higher blood glucose and circulating insulin levels suggest that they had undiagnosed type 2 diabetes prior to becoming pregnant. Type 2 diabetes is a chronic condition of insulin-resistance. I will say a little more about both types in Chapter 3 but this book is mainly discussing the much more common situation of the temporary insulin-resistance of pregnancy causing hyperglycaemia of varying degrees, which is commonly known as Gestational Diabetes Mellitus or GDM.

GDM might even be better described as hyperglycaemia of pregnancy. There is no clear blood glucose level or cut-off point at which women can be diagnosed as having 'gestational diabetes'. Normal blood glucose levels vary a little from person to person. However, we do know that the higher a pregnant woman's blood glucose levels, the greater chance of some pregnancy problems (see Box I below), and that there is a relationship between <u>increasing</u> blood glucose and <u>increasing</u> pregnancy problems. It is not possible to give an absolute risk or figure for any individual one of these problems – there is a <u>slightly</u> increased risk of any and all of them when your blood glucose is above normal and that risk increases as blood glucose levels increase. I am going to look more at this issue of risk in a few paragraphs further on where I discuss the HAPO Study.

Box 1 : Complications associated with GDM/hyperglycaemia during pregnancy

MOTHER	BABY
• Pre-eclampsia • Caesarean section • High blood pressure • Forceps/vacuum birth • Type 2 diabetes in later life • Metabolic syndrome in later life (abnormal glucose tolerance, abdominal obesity, high cholesterol, high blood pressure) which is strongly associated with cardiovascular disease.	• Macrosomia (large baby → 4kg or 8lbs 13oz) • Preterm birth (before 37 weeks) • Shoulder dystocia (baby's shoulder wedged tightly in pelvis → birth impeded) • Birth injury • Hypoglycaemia (Blood glucose <2.2mmol/L) • Newborn jaundice • Admission to neonatal special care • Still birth • Neonatal death (baby dies within the first month of life) • Obesity in later life • Type 2 diabetes in later life

So GDM is really a label used to denote blood glucose levels that correlate with increased rates of certain poorer outcomes of pregnancy, but diagnostic levels can change over time and in different places. In this sense, it is not a 'disease', but more of an indicator for more frequent care and intervention to try to reduce glucose levels and to reduce the risk of having the problems listed in Box 1 (many of these problems are discussed in more depth in Chapters 4 and 5).

The blood glucose levels at which GDM is diagnosed by the maternity services may have changed since your last pregnancy; they have certainly changed since your mother was pregnant with you. They may even differ between hospitals and do differ between countries; I write about this in some detail in Chapter 3. You could say that the thresholds for diagnosis are somewhat arbitrary; however, that does not mean that 'GDM' is not a problem. It does mean that people may interpret the problem differently depending on how they view the outcomes associated with increased glucose levels – as problematic or risky or acceptable or less important than other issues.

To understand the background to all this, it is helpful to look at an important study called HAPO – The **H**yperglycaemia and **A**dverse **P**regnancy **O**utcomes study (The HAPO Study Cooperative Research Group, 2008). HAPO consisted of a large group of pregnant women (over 25,000) from 9 countries who were tested with a 2-hour 75g **oral glucose tolerance test** (**OGTT**) and were then followed through pregnancy with their birth outcomes recorded. (What an OGTT is and how it is done is discussed in the next chapter.)

The HAPO study showed that a range of adverse pregnancy outcomes increased proportionally in relation to blood glucose levels measured at the OGTT, and this confirmed previous research findings that, as blood glucose levels increased, birthweight and fetal **hyperinsulinaemia**[3] also increased proportionally (Moses *et al.*, 1995).

An increase in other complications and interventions was also shown to be statistically significant in relation to maternal blood glucose levels but less so with birth weight and fetal insulin levels. These are: **pre-eclampsia**, caesarean section, **birth injuries** and **hypoglycaemia** (low blood glucose) in the newborn baby.

The HAPO study did not determine at what point increasing blood glucose levels in pregnancy should be called Gestational Diabetes; it simply presented the increasing rates of these complications associated with those levels. Other organisations have set the blood glucose levels at which Gestational Diabetes is diagnosed (e.g. **The International Diabetes in Pregnancy Study Group** or **IADPSG, The World Health Organisation** or **WHO** and **The National Institute for Health and Care Excellence** or **NICE**) and this is discussed in Chapter 2.

However, it is not a lot of use being able to identify women with GDM unless treatment offered to those women actually reduces the problems associated with their GDM. If there is no good treatment to help them and their babies, then testing for and diagnosing GDM would simply make a lot of people anxious and concerned, cost money and benefit nobody. Can treatment reduce the number of women and babies experiencing the problems listed in Box 1?

---

3 This is measured by the amount of C-peptide in cord blood, C-peptide being a blood marker of high insulin levels. A fetus exposed to high levels of glucose will produce more insulin to cope with this, and insulin is a sort of growth hormone so the fetus gets bigger and lays down more fat.

The World Health Organisation (WHO, 2013) undertook a **systematic review** of research into the association between increasing levels of blood glucose in pregnant women and the outcomes of their pregnancies and the effectiveness of treatment. The WHO, like HAPO, concluded that women with hyperglycaemia detected during pregnancy are at greater risk for adverse pregnancy outcomes, most notably, **macrosomia** of the newborn (large babies) and **pre-eclampsia**. Treatment of hyperglycaemia or GDM, through lifestyle and dietary changes or drugs or insulin, was found to be effective in reducing **macrosomia, shoulder dystocia** and **pre-eclampsia/ hypertensive disorders in pregnancy**, and **hypoglycaemia** in the baby. The WHO concluded that:

The risk reduction for these outcomes is in general large, the number needed to treat is low, and the quality of evidence is adequate to justify treatment of GDM. (WHO, 2013, p.3)

So, the general opinion amongst health professionals is that it is worth women being tested for GDM because there are treatments available that are known to reduce the incidence of some problems. (Treatments are discussed in Chapter 4.) However, as in all health matters, it is difficult to apply conclusions arising from the study of large populations to individuals, and I discuss what being tested and treated for GDM may mean for you as an individual and a family in Chapter 2.

Preventing GDM when you are already pregnant – the research so far

Some research has been done to see if interventions during early pregnancy can reduce the rate of GDM amongst women at risk (e.g.

those with higher BMIs). Overall, they have not found much evidence that intervention prevents GDM in women once they are pregnant.

Lifestyle changes (diet and exercise)

A number of studies have looked at preventing GDM through lifestyle change during pregnancy and the picture is somewhat mixed. One review concluded that diet interventions alone were associated with an overall 33% reduction in risk of GDM, whilst diet and exercise interventions in combination were not associated with any reduction

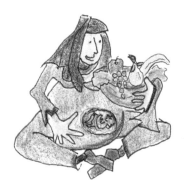

in GDM rates (Rogozinska *et al.*, 2015). However, another review showed an overall reduction in risk of GDM of 31% with physical activity interventions (Sanabria-Martínez *et al.*, 2015). Neither the UPBEAT Study in the UK (Poston *et al.*, 2015) nor the DALI Study across 11 centres in Europe (Simmons, 2016) found any reduction in GDM rates from their various lifestyle interventions (exercise, diet and combined) even when **gestational weight gain** was restricted, though both of these studies measured outcomes from lifestyle interventions that started after the first three months of pregnancy.

However, an extensive **systematic review** (looking at 29 trials involving 11,500 women) showed that there is a potentially very strong impact (80% reduction in GDM) if lifestyle intervention is started before 15 weeks' gestation, whilst intervention later during pregnancy is less effective (18% reduction in GDM) (Song *et al.*, 2016). On the other hand, the latest review of nutritional interventions concluded that *no strong conclusion can be drawn with regard to the best intervention for the prevention of GDM* (Donaza-Ezcurra et al., 2017).

So you can see that some of the studies have found dietary changes during pregnancy to be beneficial, others have found increasing physical activity during pregnancy to be helpful, and others have found neither to be of help in preventing GDM when started later in pregnancy! But it does look like changes in lifestyle (diet and activity) early in pregnancy is beneficial (Song et al., 2016).

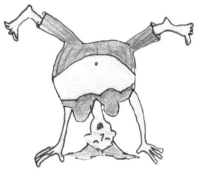

There is also increasing evidence that gaining too much weight in pregnancy (more than 13–15kg) is not good in terms of increased babies' birthweights, caesarean section and GDM rates, and longer term BMIs (Siega-Riz et al., 2009; Beyerlein et al., 2011). In addition, eating a healthy diet[4] has many benefits to you and your baby regardless of any impact on GDM, and pregnancy is a good time to look closely at what you eat and make changes.

It is not yet known whether restricting **gestational weight gain** through lifestyle changes during pregnancy has any longer-term benefit (such as reducing rates of later type 2 diabetes, or reducing obesity rates in the children). It appears from studies that restricting weight gain during pregnancy to 5 to 8kg, or even less than 5kg in overweight or obese women, is not associated with any problems for them or

---

4 A healthy diet is defined here as small, regular nutritious meals consisting of high fibre and wholefoods, plenty of protein and non-starchy vegetables and fruit, with very little or no sugar.

their babies (Simmons, 2016). If you are **not** overweight or obese, it is not known whether restricting weight gain to this extent is safe or beneficial. Most studies done on GDM prevention recruit women with higher BMIs, and very little is known about GDM in women with lower BMIs.

What is not known but currently being explored, is whether lifestyle change leading to weight loss *before* pregnancy means there will be less risk of developing GDM. Given that lifestyle change and weight loss is known to prevent or even reverse type 2 diabetes (see Chapter 6), this is a promising area to research as a similar approach may be successful in preventing GDM. Also, given that GDM is strongly associated with weight and BMI, then any reduction in these is likely to lower the risk of GDM.

Vitamin D supplementation
Women with lower levels of Vitamin D have been found to be more likely to develop GDM than women with higher levels. Also, women are more likely to be diagnosed with GDM in the summer than in the winter (i.e. they have become pregnant when Vitamin D stores are at their lowest in the winter). Vitamin D is mainly made by the action of sunlight on the skin and plays an important role in the metabolism of calcium. In particular, dark-skinned women living in less sunny climates and women who keep themselves covered up when out-of-doors, tend to have lower levels of Vitamin D and may be deficient in Vitamin D. Heavy use of sun-screen can also lead to lower Vitamin D levels as the sun is unable to act on the skin to make sufficient Vitamin D. Also the further north you live, the more likely you are to be short of Vitamin D, especially during winter months. And just to make it even harder to maintain good levels of Vitamin D, the bigger you are, the more likely you are to be short of Vitamin D.

We get a small amount of Vitamin D from our diet (e.g. oily fish, eggs, margarine, liver, cheese, butter and full-fat milk) but the vast majority is obtained through the exposure of skin to direct sunlight (20 to 30 minutes a day is usually enough for most people with paler skin and the sun doesn't have to be shining, but you may need to be out for longer if it is cloudy or you have darker skin[5]. Pregnancy and pre-pregnancy vitamin supplements all contain Vitamin D, as do Healthy Start Vitamins provided by the UK Department of Health.

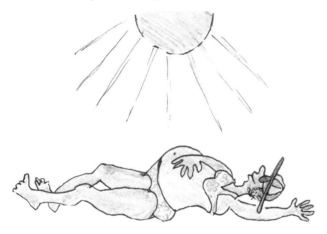

Because of a theoretical association of lower Vitamin D with GDM (and type 2 diabetes), extra Vitamin D has been given to women in research studies to see if it reduces the rate of GDM. However, this has not been shown to have any effect, so whilst you may want to make sure you have adequate exposure to sunlight and take the recommended daily amount (10 mcg/400 international units a day) to maintain general health, there is no evidence that taking any extra Vitamin D will prevent GDM (De-Regil et al., 2016; Corcoy, 2015).

---

5 For more information, see *https://www.vitamindcouncil.org/about-vitamin-d/ how-do-i-get-the-vitamin-d-my-body-needs/*

You can ask to have your Vitamin D levels tested (a blood test). Vitamin D is important for many aspects of our health, including our mental health, so supplements can be prescribed if your levels are low, though we still know relatively little about the benefits of supplementation during pregnancy (De-Regil et al., 2016).

Drugs

The EMPOWaR study looked at metformin and compared metformin to a placebo tablet in overweight, non-diabetic, pregnant women but found it had no effect on a range of outcomes, including GDM rates (Chiswick et al., 2015), though there was some improvement in plasma glucose levels and insulin sensitivity in the treatment (metformin) group. Metformin was taken from 12-16 weeks gestation until birth. Similar findings but with reduced weight gain during pregnancy were reported by the MOP (Metformin in Obese Pregnancy) Study (Syngelaki et al., 2016).

Alternatives

Acupuncture has been found to improve glucose tolerance and insulin-sensitivity in studies on rats (Chang et al., 2006). I am not aware of any study showing that acupuncture has the same effect on humans although practitioners of Traditional Chinese Medicine may be in a better position to advise on this.

Astralagus ('huang qi' in Chinese) is a plant native to Asia, the root of which is widely used in Chinese medicine. In a study reported from China, women were treated with either insulin only or insulin and astralagus for GDM (there was no group that was untreated). Those who were treated with insulin and astralagus achieved better blood glucose control than those on insulin alone. The authors suggest that astralagus *may play a role in the prevention and treatment of GDM*

(Liang et al., 2009). Astralagus is widely available as a supplement in the UK, but always be cautious when exploring the use of Chinese medicines as they can be very potent, and so I recommend consulting with a qualified practitioner of Chinese Traditional Medicine.

Cinnamon is another alternative for preventing or treating GDM that you may come across on the Internet. Cinnamon contains polyphenols that are thought to improve insulin sensitivity or function. Cinnamon can be dissolved in hot water and taken as a drink, or sprinkled on toast. Some research has been carried out on its effects on glucose tolerance in type 2 diabetes (**NOT** GDM) with mixed findings – it may have some benefits but also be harmful to anyone with impaired liver function (Allen et al., 2013).

If you do want to consider alternative approaches, as with any intervention, it is important to do your research and to consider asking for guidance from a qualified practitioner. Acupuncture, herbs, homeopathy, probiotics and tissue salts are all reported to have helped some women – look on the internet for information and/or consult your complementary therapist.

(For information about prevention of Type 2 diabetes after GDM or recurrence of GDM in future pregnancies, please see Chapter 6.)

Chapter 2:
Having the test for GDM - is it for you?

Blood tests for gestational diabetes and diabetes

There are a number of blood tests used to screen for, test for and diagnose GDM and diabetes. Screening tests are those which identify people whose chance of having a condition is greater than X. Diagnostic tests are those which determine whether or not a condition is actually present.

- **Random Blood Glucose (RBG)** or more correctly **Random Plasma Glucose (RPG)**

This is exactly as it sounds – blood taken at any time of day or in relation to meals. It may be offered alongside other tests by your community midwife at your first visit for antenatal care.

RPG is not a test to diagnose GDM but is a screening test often offered at the first antenatal visit. Its purpose is to identify women who may have high blood glucose at that stage and to offer them more specific tests earlier in pregnancy than they might otherwise be offered. You can have a high RPG result yet NOT have any form of diabetes at all (called a false-positive result) or, less commonly, you can have a normal RPG but have underlying high glucose levels (called a false-negative result).

If your result is more than 7mmol/L, you will be offered an early Oral Glucose Tolerance Test or OGTT (see below).

- **Fasting Blood Glucose (FBG)** or more correctly **Fasting Plasma Glucose (FPG)**

This is when blood is taken following a period of fasting, usually in the morning after having nothing to eat or drink (other than sips of water) overnight. It also forms part of the **Oral Glucose Tolerance Test (OGTT)** (see below) but can be done as a stand-alone test.

- **Glucose Challenge Test (GCT)**

This is a non-fasting test which measures the level of blood sugar after you have had a drink which contains a specific amount of glucose (50 grams). An hour later a blood test is done to check your plasma glucose level.

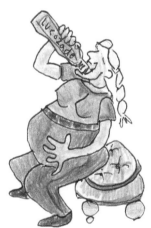

The GCT may be offered by your community midwife in the UK between 24 and 28 weeks of pregnancy, using a drink that provides 50g glucose (usually 273mls of Lucozade Original™)[6]. You should have nothing to eat or drink during the hour's wait between drinking the glucose drink and your blood being taken, as this would affect the test result. For some women the drink is nauseating, particularly if they cannot eat for an hour after drinking it.

The GCT is, like the Random Plasma Glucose (RPG) above, a screening test to determine who may be offered an OGTT (see below). It can also, like the RPG, give false positive results (i.e. your result can be high without you having any form of diabetes).

If your GCT result is greater than 7.8mmol/L, you will be offered an oral Glucose Tolerance Test. This higher-level threshold is because the

---

6 I am not mentioning this brand to favour it, but because it is the only widely available glucose drink manufactured with consistently accurate glucose content, hence why it is commonly used for these tests.

GCT is testing how your body dealt with the glucose drink that you had an hour earlier.

- **Oral Glucose Tolerance Test (OGTT)**

This is the main diagnostic test for GDM and is usually done around or before 28 weeks gestation.

There is evidence that the increased fetal growth, which the identification and treatment of GDM is aiming to prevent, actually begins before 28 weeks, and this is particularly so for women with BMIs of 30 or above (Sovio *et al.*, 2016). Sovio and colleagues found that the incidence of increased fetal growth was already observed by 20 weeks among women classified as obese. They recommend that screening and intervention for GDM is carried out before 20 weeks for women with higher BMIs, for treatment to have a positive impact on the later health of babies. If you have a higher BMI and want to be screened for GDM, you may want to discuss earlier testing with your midwife or doctor. Or, if you have other risk factors for GDM (see the list below) and want screening, you may want to ask for this to be done earlier than 28 weeks so that any treatment is more effective in preventing your baby growing so large.

The OGTT involves fasting overnight, having a fasting plasma glucose test, then drinking a known amount of glucose (usually 75g taken either as water with glucose powder dissolved in it or 410mls[7] Lucozade Original™), and having blood taken one hour and two hours after finishing the drink. (Most women prefer Lucozade Original™ to the glucose powder drink.)

---

7 The glucose content of Lucozade Original™ is being reduced in 2017 so these volumes may change.

Plasma is one of the constituents of blood,. and this is what is tested when your blood reaches the laboratory. I will usually refer to **plasma glucose** when discussing tests and results done in a laboratory from now on.

Being offered a test for gestational diabetes in pregnancy

You may be offered a test, usually an **OGTT**, for gestational diabetes (GDM) for a variety of reasons:

* You have had gestational diabetes in an earlier pregnancy (an OGTT is normally offered earlier at around 16 weeks gestation if you have had GDM in the past). If this early OGTT is normal, you will be offered a repeat OGTT at 24-28 weeks of pregnancy;
* Your BMI is 30 or higher;
* You have a first-degree blood relative (parent or sibling) with type 1 or type 2 diabetes;
* Your ethnic origin is African-Caribbean, South Asian, Chinese or Middle Eastern [or, Hispanic, or Aboriginal, Melanesian or Maori];
* You have previously had a baby weighing 4.5kg (10 lbs) or more;
* You have had a random plasma glucose result of greater than 7.0mmol/L (see above);
* You have had a glucose challenge test with a result greater than 7.8mmol/L (see above);
* There is a lot of amniotic fluid around your baby. This is called **polyhydramnios** and it is more common with diabetes or GDM;
* Your baby feels large and is estimated to weigh above the 97th percentile on ultrasound scan. This means that he or she is thought to be in the largest 3% (approx 1 in 30) of babies at the same week of pregnancy;

* Your baby's abdomen measures more than the 97th percentile on ultrasound scan. This means that his or her tummy is thought to be in the largest 3% (approx 1 in 30) of babies' tummies at the same week of pregnancy;

* You report symptoms that suggest you may have high plasma glucose levels (usually excessive thirst or needing to drink frequently);

* Your routine antenatal urine dipstick test has shown the presence of a significant amount of glucose.

Women who fall into any category on this list are known to be at increased risk of developing GDM (NICE, 2015). Other risk factors for GDM are **polycystic ovary syndrome**, twin or multiple babies' pregnancy, and being older, e.g. over 35 years, and some maternity units may routinely add these factors to the list above. You should also be offered a test if you are on anti-retroviral (HIV) drugs, long-term steroid therapy, post-transplant drugs or certain anti-psychotic drugs (e.g. quetiapine), as all these are associated with a greater likelihood of GDM.

A few units offer <u>all</u> women testing for GDM because they serve an area with a large population from black and minority ethnic groups, who have a higher incidence of GDM. However, testing is expensive and time-consuming so the number of units doing this is small as it would not be deemed cost-effective in many areas.

Nevertheless, nearly half of women diagnosed with GDM do not have any of these risk factors and many that do have them do not develop GDM (Stewart, 2014). It is just *more likely* that you will develop GDM with these factors than if you do not have them.

What tests are offered?

Any of the tests described above may be offered to you but the diagnostic test for GDM is the Oral Glucose Tolerance Test (OGTT). The others are only screening tests informing health care professionals which women they should be offering an OGTT to, and for which women it is probably not indicated. Only the OGTT can provide the basis for a diagnosis of GDM.

Deciding whether to have a blood test for GDM

The only person who has the right to decide what tests she does or does not accept in pregnancy is the pregnant woman herself. Whether or not you accept a test for GDM is entirely your decision and yours alone, even if you have a higher chance of developing GDM. Even though **NICE** recommends screening for GDM during pregnancy, it is still your decision as to whether or not to have any test offered. You may want to think about your own personal risk factors first, such as BMI, ethnic background, family history of diabetes, previous baby weights and so on. Other things to consider are whether you would accept the treatments on offer or find the additional support helpful (Chapter 4), and how it may affect your birth choices (listed in Box 2 and discussed below).

If the result of the OGGT test shows that you have plasma glucose levels in the GDM range, this will affect what you are offered, and the advice given to you for the rest of your pregnancy in a number of ways. How you relate to these interventions will be personal – you may welcome all or some of them. You may not like the thought of any of the interventions, but decide to be tested just to be certain. On the other hand, the interventions may be unacceptable to you because they do not accord with your beliefs, or your hopes and aspirations for this pregnancy and birth, and you decline the test because a positive test result would cause you distress and anxiety.

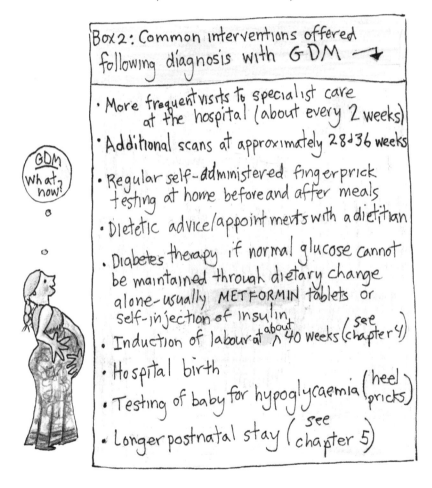

Box 2: Common interventions offered following diagnosis with GDM →

- More frequent visits to specialist care at the hospital (about every 2 weeks)
- Additional scans at approximately 28 & 36 weeks
- Regular self-administered fingerprick testing at home before and after meals
- Dietetic advice/appointments with a dietitian
- Diabetes therapy if normal glucose cannot be maintained through dietary change alone – usually METFORMIN tablets or self-injection of insulin
- Induction of labour at about 40 weeks (see chapter 4)
- Hospital birth
- Testing of baby for hypoglycaemia (heel pricks)
- Longer postnatal stay (see chapter 5)

How you feel about the package of care that is offered to women receiving a positive OGTT test result will depend very much on your previous experiences, your plans and their importance to you, your beliefs and values, and those of the people close to you. What is important is that you are aware of the likely consequences of a positive result before you have the test. If you are diagnosed with GDM following an OGTT, it is likely that you will come under pressure to accept these interventions, and you will have to make decisions about each and every one of them.

You will want to weigh up the risks of GDM for you and your baby (see above and in the next chapter), the risks of the interventions on offer (such as induction of labour[8], additional ultrasound scans[9]), and what alternatives may be available to you if you receive a positive result. To what extent would having support from your partner, your family and your friends about your decision to accept or to decline the test be valuable to you?

Of course, if you do have the test and it comes back as negative, that is within the normal range, you will probably feel relieved. It does not, however, mean that you will definitely not have any of the complications associated with GDM. It simply means that the likelihood of, say, a large baby or caesarean section are less for someone with normal plasma glucose levels than they are for another woman with higher plasma glucose levels.

There are further issues raised by the fact that there are differing diagnostic criteria in use that you need to be aware of when making your decision about whether to consent to an OGTT for GDM. I discuss this in detail in Chapter 3.

---

8 See AIMS book *Inducing Labour: Making Informed Decisions* by S. Wickham, listed in References.

9 See AIMS book *Ultrasound? Unsound* by B. Lawrence Beech and J. Robinson, listed in References.

Having the test for GDM: going for an OGTT

One of the effects of a well-balanced healthy diet is to keep blood glucose relatively stable. It is obvious that what you eat in the day or two before the test can affect the result to some degree. Diabetes UK has some very good information on how to choose a healthy low carbohydrate diet, and meal and snack suggestions on its website: *www.diabetes.org.uk/Guide-to-diabetes/Managing-your-diabetes/Healthy-eating*. In the 3 or 4 days before the test, eating a healthy diet of plenty of green vegetables, protein such as meat or fish or pulses, nuts and wholegrains, cutting out as much sugary food and refined carbohydrates (white bread and pasta, biscuits, cakes and sweets and sugary drinks), and taking moderate daily exercise for at least 30 minutes will give you a better chance of having a normal OGTT result as it will optimise your blood glucose levels prior to the test. However, it is debatable how desirable it is to 'trick' any test you go for, so do consider this point if a 'healthy diet' is very different from your usual diet. Masking your true blood glucose picture temporarily for the test will not lower the likelihood of the problems if your usual blood glucose is higher. You should assess this advice (which is found in many discussions on the Internet) on an individual basis, and in relation to your eating habits.

You will need to have nothing to eat or drink (other than occasional sips of water if very thirsty or to take medication) from the previous evening (your midwife can advise you more precisely depending on the time of your OGTT appointment, but 10pm is often the time given from which to fast if your OGTT appointment is between 8.30 and 9.30 the following morning). You should refrain from taking any antacids (such as Gaviscon, Rennies etc) during this period.

If you have had bariatric surgery (a gastric bypass or sleeve or other similar technique), then you should not have an OGTT even if you fall into one or more of the categories listed above on pages 27/28. This is because of the danger of 'rebound' hypoglycaemia or low blood sugar, what your doctor may have described to you as 'dumping'. One or more of the other tests not requiring you to drink a bolus of glucose can be offered instead.

The OGTT normally takes TWO HOURS so take something to read and try to get any toddlers looked after. And remember that clinic waiting rooms are not very comfortable and, as you should not walk around much during an OGTT (because it affects the accuracy of the result), you may want to take a cushion to sit on! You should also not smoke during the test as this would also affect the result.

It is possible to have the test performed at home but few community midwifery services have the capacity to offer this. Also, the samples have to be processed in the laboratory promptly so this is an added difficulty. Once fasting bloods have been taken, you will be offered a glucose drink with a known amount of glucose in it. Remember, you may be thirsty and want to gulp it down, but your pregnancy may make you feel nauseous if you drink too quickly. Take your time, especially if it is a fizzy drink. You have five minutes to drink it so do take it slowly – 410 mls is nearly a pint so it is quite a big drink! If you know you have trouble keeping fizzy drinks down, ask the person doing the test to pour the drink out on arrival so that it is a little flatter by the time you drink it. If you vomit any of the drink at any time during the test (whilst you are drinking it or afterwards), the test will have to be cancelled and rearranged.

The person taking the blood will note the time you finish the drink, and take blood at a set interval after that time (either at 60 and 120 minutes or just at 120 minutes), so remember not to go off to the loo when those times are coming up, as delay in taking the one- and two-hour bloods will affect the result.

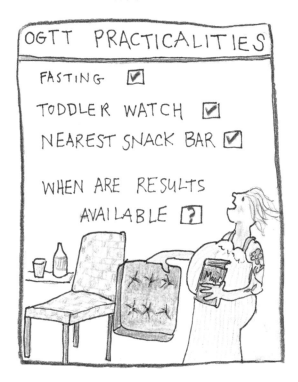

The OGTT requires a needle to be inserted into your arm two or three times (depending on whether or not the hospital tests a 60-minute sample). If you are due to have other blood tests around the same time, ask your midwife when she is arranging the OGTT, or whoever is doing it, to see if they can be done at the same time (any number of bottles of blood for tests can be taken on one needle-insertion).

Once the two hours is over and all the blood taken, have a drink and a snack or a meal before you make any attempt to travel – take some food and drink with you if you can, or ask where the nearest snack bar or restaurant is if you are in an unfamiliar part of the hospital and need to buy something. If you are feeling at all faint, tell the staff and ask for help. Most people do feel OK after an OGTT but pregnancy can be a time when your body reacts more than usual to not eating for a while.

Before you leave, make sure you know what the process and likely time-scale is for you to receive the results.

Women's Experiences

I was routinely tested for GDM with a 2 hour glucose test (due to maternal family ethnicity) with my first daughter and was negative. Though, unfortunately, the test was positive when pregnant with my second daughter... I was very borderline and even asked to be re-tested as I was surprised. Unfortunately, the doctor didn't agree to a re-test. **Stacey, GDM with second baby**

I had glucose in my urine at two midwife appointments (at home) so I was sent for an OGTT. I remember it being quite automatic, I don't remember thinking too much about it, I think partly because it never even crossed my mind I would actually have GDM. It definitely wasn't put to me as a choice with any pros/cons/consequences presented. At that stage in pregnancy (about 34 weeks) I wasn't feeling nauseous at all and didn't find the test itself too onerous (this was my first baby so no childcare issues). Although it isn't pleasant, obviously. I was devastated by the consequences of having the test. The diagnosis itself was not a huge issue for me (I was grateful to be aware of it) and I was able to control it easily and quickly with my diet. But the GDM label I had on my maternity notes and the orange sheets in them, as a consequence of being diagnosed, were devastating.

When I was pregnant with my second baby I went to my booking in at 10 weeks and had glucose in my urine again. The (kind) midwife looked at her chart and said I would be referred to the diabetes clinic. I declined and said I would just test my blood sugars myself. If I kept them in range, I was comfortable I was 'low risk'. I followed a strict diet and my blood sugar was fine the whole pregnancy. I was 'offered' an OGTT several times but it was not pressed upon me at all. I made it clear I considered it completely pointless considering I was already testing my blood sugars. Since this is what is done anyway AFTER an OGTT it would have made no sense to have one in my opinion. I'm not even sure how well they reflect what is really going on in your body anyway? But maybe it is the best diagnostic tool available (or maybe the cheapest). At 28 weeks we moved house and I signed up to the home birth team at the new hospital. The midwife was AMAZING. I saw only her for the rest of my pregnancy. She was totally supportive of me. She did need to do a risk assessment to say that I had declined an OGTT and it was my choice to have a homebirth but that didn't bother me at all. My daughter was born at home at 41+4 weeks, 8lbs 5oz.

I have recently had a 3rd baby and I again took responsibility for my own blood sugars and did not have the OGTT. Although this time I did not test much – I ate very carefully from 5 weeks pregnant, and did some random blood sugar tests as we went along. I went for the Michel Odent approach – eat a great diet (and I was really careful), and trust your body. I was an expert in a low GI diet by this point, and I did stick to that carefully. This was an easy, healthy and happy pregnancy and third baby was born at home in water. **Lisa, had GDM with first baby, chose not to have OGTT with second and third babies**

When I became pregnant again just over a year later, I knew I would do things differently and I did. I used the One to One Midwives service, and confident in the care of my named midwife, I chose not to have an OGTT. I gave birth to my second son, who weighed 7lbs 14oz at 40 weeks, at home in water. I was fortunate that I'd read widely on the subject and felt confident enough with the support of my midwife to fight for the pregnancy and birth I wanted but I'm aware that this won't be the case for all women. It should be and I wish it was. **Sophie, had GDM with first baby but chose not to be tested with second baby**

The first time I was tested because a distant relative had diabetes and it turned out I shouldn't have been. Wasn't really given a choice was just told that I needed it. I had the type of test where I had to drink a drink and wait for 2 hours to have a blood test. I took some time off work, and a good book, and it was no trouble. The second time I wasn't given the test at 28 weeks as the family history wasn't close enough. I constantly had traces of glucose in my urine so was finally tested at about 35 weeks. In hindsight, I should have been tested a lot earlier, again not a choice more of a necessity. I got someone to look after my daughter while I went for the test as it was too long to take her with me; it would take around 2.5 hours. Not eating was a bit of a struggle when pregnant but for the right reasons. The drink wasn't particularly nice so I am glad that it is just a simple blood test now (at my GP's each year). The waiting around was a bit annoying as you weren't allowed to leave and come back. **Joanna, GDM with second baby**

I wouldn't say I was really aware of there being a choice over having the test. That said, knowing if I had GDM that may cause issues, then the 'choice' was quite simple. I had the oral solution drink and didn't find it that bad at all. The waiting around was a pain, with very little to do in a dull waiting room that ironically holds 2 vending machines full of chocolate and crisps!! I seem to remember also having a blood test before and after the 2 hours had lapsed and then I was free to go. The appointment *time was an absolute pain and did mean that I was beyond starving and therefore didn't feel too great, but was absolutely fine after I'd eaten.* **Nicola, GDM with first baby**

With regards to the option for a OGTT, I don't believe I felt I had an option, but I knew in my gut that I had the condition so I knew I needed to be tested. For the actual procedure, fasting from the night before was tough, particularly as I had sickness through the pregnancy and needed to eat frequently to stop being sick so I did spend the time of the test feeling a bit rough, but the actual drink itself wasn't too bad. Another lady had her OGTT at the same session as me so we had a good chat and the time just flew by. **Nicki, GDM with first baby**

I developed gestational diabetes during my second pregnancy (but not my first or third). I was routinely tested because my father has diabetes, meaning that my risk was higher; I had not had any noticeable symptoms. I did not question whether the test (OGTT) was necessary, I never felt as though I had an option about the OGTT, it was booked in for me without me ever being asked if I wanted it, I was just told about it. I was also never given any options for other tests other than the OGTT. The test itself was fine.

During my third pregnancy (having had GDM in my second but not my first pregnancy), I did consider refusing the test because being labelled as diabetic had caused me more problems in my second pregnancy than actually managing my blood sugars. I considered just going on the same diet and not actually finding out but in the end I decided that I wanted to know. However, had I been diabetic again then I was not going to go to the regular diabetes clinic again because I had found it so unpleasant and stressful. Previously, I wasn't told much about the test before I went - I was given a one-page information sheet which just covered practicalities about where to report to when and about not eating, etc. I wasn't told anything about what they were actually testing, what the results could be and what result would mean that I was 'diabetic' – I later discovered *that the threshold for being labelled as diabetic is not the same in all hospitals which concerned me. I have a friend who did refuse the test because she was referred to it based on her BMI being over a particular number. However, she is healthy, fit and very tall so she didn't feel that, in her instance, her BMI put her at higher risk. I have had the OGTT 5 times now (including postnatal tests) so I became very used to the test itself. I was lucky that the dates I was given fell on work days so my older children were already due to be in nursery and childcare was not an issue and my work are reasonable and understanding. If it had fallen on a non-work day I'm not sure what I would have done, I would have tried to move it to a work day, but if that wasn't possible it would have been very difficult for me because we were told not to bring children to the test, and I don't have any family nearby so childcare would have been an issue. The actual test was okay, I didn't enjoy not eating and I think I had some nausea (especially when I was tested earlier in my third pregnancy), but nothing too bad. I don't like Lucozade so again didn't enjoy having to drink it but I didn't find it that big a deal. In my second. and third pregnancies, getting to sit and do nothing for a couple of hours was a bonus! I distinctly remember, though, the person who took my blood telling me that if I was diabetic that I would be induced early – not that I would have this option or that that was their advice but that it would happen. **Rebecca, GDM with second baby but not first or third***

*I went for my glucose test whilst pregnant but didn't expect to get a positive result. When having my daughter 4½ years ago, I didn't get GDM so I never expected to get it next time round. It always played on my mind that I may have it because my father sadly passed away from uncontrolled diabetes 17 years ago at the age of 63. I have a BMI of 30 and am 39 years old so I knew in this pregnancy I was higher risk than before. When I took the glucose test, I didn't realise the full impact it would take on my emotions and pregnancy. **Zoe, GDM with second baby***

I was diagnosed with GD early on in my third pregnancy, at 12 weeks. I found the GTT test to be particularly difficult to do while pregnant and would have preferred the option of monitoring my blood sugar levels before and after a meal like some hospitals offer. **Suzanna, GDM with third baby**

Chapter 3:
Making sense of the test results

Getting the results

These are available 24 to 72 hours after the test, and are usually sent to you by letter if normal and by phone and/or letter if they fall within the range for a diagnosis of GDM. Depending on your blood results, you will either be found to have 'normal' plasma glucose levels, or be told that you have gestational diabetes, or you may be diagnosed with Type 2 diabetes. This latter scenario is becoming more common in younger people and you will almost certainly have had the diabetes before the pregnancy; the extra tests during pregnancy have just brought it to light.

Diabetes Mellitus: being diagnosed with diabetes for the first time when you are pregnant

According to the WHO (2013), diabetes should be diagnosed in pregnancy (as at other times) if one or more of the following are found:

Fasting plasma glucose greater or equal to 7.0mmol/L.
2-hour plasma glucose greater or equal to 11.1mmol/L following a 75g oral glucose load.
Random plasma glucose greater or equal to 11.1mmol/L in the presence of diabetes symptoms.

If blood test results are in the ranges above, then further investigations will determine what type of diabetes is present; it will almost always be either Type 1 or Type 2 Diabetes Mellitus.

Diabetes symptoms include:

* Going to the toilet a lot, especially at night
* Being really thirsty
* Feeling more tired than usual
* Losing weight without trying to (less likely in pregnancy)
* Genital itching or thrush
* Cuts and wounds take longer to heal
* Blurred vision

Type 1 Diabetes Mellitus is an auto-immune condition where the insulin-producing ß (beta) cells in the pancreas stop functioning. Its cause is unknown and it is a lifelong condition requiring the administration of insulin supplements by sub-cutaneous injection or continuous pump infusion to maintain cell-function and life. Whilst it usually arises during childhood or adolescence, it can occur at any time and a very small number of women are diagnosed with diabetes for the first time when they are pregnant. Type 1 diabetes can be differentiated from type 2 diabetes by the presence of particular antibodies in the blood.

A specialist diabetes team consisting of a diabetologist, diabetes specialist nurse and dietitian will help you manage your diabetes and there are good systems in place in most areas enabling you to keep in touch with them for support and advice by telephone, email, social media, and face-to-face appointments.

Type 2 Diabetes Mellitus is where your body doesn't produce enough insulin to meet its requirements, usually due to increased insulin resistance secondary to increased weight and fat deposits, but also due to a variety of other reasons. In type 2 diabetes, there is often a high amount of insulin in the blood, whereas in type 1 diabetes, insulin is almost absent. You will usually be helped to manage your type 2 diabetes in the community, by your GP and practice nurse, once your baby has been born. This is usually initially managed by **metformin** tablets and lifestyle changes, though insulin is often required during pregnancy.

For further information on Types 1 and 2 diabetes mellitus, please visit the Diabetes UK website, *www.diabetes.org.uk.*

Being told you have any form of diabetes will almost certainly be a bit of a shock and many women do feel very upset on receiving the news. In the introduction to this book I made a number of suggestions about talking to other women who have received the same diagnosis, and there are further suggestions of sources of help and support in the section on e-resources at the end of this book. Taking some time to talk through the issues and how you are feeling with someone can be very helpful, whether face-to-face, by telephone or email.

Being diagnosed with gestational diabetes mellitus (GDM) during pregnancy

In many ways, this is a bit more complicated than being diagnosed with diabetes itself. What you are actually being diagnosed with is a level of plasma glucose or hyperglycaemia, associated with a higher risk of an adverse outcome, as listed in Box 1 (page 14). Also, remember there are different diagnostic criteria in use in different hospitals and different countries. So you may be told you have GDM in one place, which uses one set of criteria, when you would be told you do not have GDM in another place that uses a different set of criteria, on the same OGTT results!

The results used to determine the cut-off for GDM diagnosis can be set at different risk levels (or risk ratios) of the things listed in Box 1. A table of the various OGTT GDM diagnostic levels can be found in Box 3.

Box 3 (All numbers are expressed in mmol/L)
(≥ means equal to or greater than   > means greater than)

Organisation	Fasting result	1 hour result	2 hour result	3 hour result
IADPSG/ WHO	≥ 5.1	≥ 10.0	≥ 8.5	N/A
NICE	≥ 5.6	N/A	≥ 7.8	N/A
ACOG	≥ 5.3	≥ 10.0	≥ 8.6	≥ 7.8
ADA	> 5.3	> 10.0	> 8.5	N/A
Your maternity provider	?	?	?	?

DIAGNOSIS OF GDM: Plasma glucose Measurements BY DIFFERENT ORGANISATIONS

For example, both the International Association of the Diabetes and Pregnancy Study Groups (**IADPSG**) and the World Health Organisation (**WHO**) criteria for GDM is an OGTT result of ≥5.1mmol/L for fasting plasma glucose and/or ≥10.0mmol/L one hour after the glucose drink and/or ≥8.5mmol/L two hours after the glucose drink of 75g glucose. You only need <u>ONE</u> measurement to be above or equal to these figures for a diagnosis of GDM. However, many UK maternity units who use the IADPSG/WHO test results nonetheless use a 5.3mmol/L cut off for the fasting result instead of 5.1mmol/L to diagnose GDM, even though they use the same one and two hour measurements as above.

How are these criteria decided? The IADPSG/WHO used the HAPO Study mentioned in Chapter 2 to establish their criteria, and they both set the diagnosis of GDM at levels where the risk (also known as 'odds ratio' - see page 50) of **macrosomia** and cord C-peptide (a marker of fetal **hyperinsulinaemia**) were increased by three-quarters (or by a ratio of 1 to 1.75). In other words, women with hyperglycaemia as defined by the IADPSG/WHO criteria were 75% more likely to experience certain problems (IADPSG Consensus Panel, 2010). For example, if we expect 10% of women with normal blood glucose to give birth to babies over 4kg (8lbs 13oz), then almost 18% (i.e. 75% more) of women with IADPSG/WHO threshold levels of hyperglycaemia would be expected to have a baby weighing more than 4kg, with that percentage rising as OGTT plasma glucose levels rise.

This is an illustration of the level of risk (usually referred to in science as odds ratios) used by the IADPSG/WHO. The coloured box at the end of this chapter discusses this in more detail but if statistics aren't your thing, don't feel obliged to read it; the key thing to remember is that we are talking about an increased chance of something happening, not the inevitability that it will. The odds are almost always that it won't happen. Taking the example above – someone not diagnosed with GDM has a 90% chance of having a baby under 4kg, and for someone diagnosed with GDM, although they have a higher chance their baby will be over 4kg, there is still an 82% chance it won't be if their glucose levels are at or just above the threshold for GDM.

In the UK, **NICE (The National Institute for Health and Care Excellence)** has set the OGTT diagnostic criteria for GDM and its recommendations are the most likely to be operating in UK maternity units (though some hospitals use the IADPSG/WHO ones).

The NICE guidelines for an OGTT in pregnancy require the fasting plasma measurement and the two hour one only. NICE criteria for GDM is a fasting plasma glucose of ≥ 5.6mmol/L or ≥ 7.8mmol/L two hours after a glucose drink of 75g glucose.

NICE did not adopt the IADPSG/WHO OGTT result levels because these levels would have resulted in almost twice as many women being diagnosed with GDM. And it was felt that this would place too great a burden on maternity services, in terms of specialist appointment time and finances because of the need for more ultrasound scans and other interventions (see Box 2 in Chapter 2). There were also concerns about the emotional cost to women of being diagnosed with GDM at these sorts of rates.

Some units in the UK have, nevertheless, adopted the IADPSG/WHO criteria in preference to the NICE criteria as there is evidence that more women with a similar raised risk of having babies weighing more than 4kg and associated emergency caesarean section will not be picked up using the NICE criteria (Meek et al, 2015). Meek and colleagues' paper shows that women with fasting plasma glucose (FPG) between 5.1 and 5.5mmol/L have very comparable levels of risk to women with FPGs of 5.6mmol/L. They recommend that the decision regarding whether to treat or not should rest with the women whose FPGs are between 5.1 and 5.5mmol/L. The authors say that adhering to the NICE guideline, and telling this group of women that they do not have

GDM, results in health care professionals misleading women and not giving them information that they need to make informed decisions.

The Born in Bradford Study, which is following 10,500 pregnant women and the babies that they gave birth to, has explored the relationship between large babies and OGTT results (all women in the study had an OGTT at around 26 weeks gestation). The study suggests that South Asian women should have more stringent GDM diagnostic criteria (fasting glucose 5.2mmol/L and 2-hr post OGTT level of 7.2mmol/L) in order to help reduce their babies' chance of increased adiposity or 'fat deposits' and cardiac problems in later life (Farrar et al., 2015).

The debate continues and it is likely that further changes to NICE guidelines will occur over the next 5 to 10 years that bring them closer to or adopting the IADPSG/WHO criteria for GDM, or ethnicity-specific criteria. Meanwhile different countries, maternity units, and even individual health care professionals, are using different cut-off points to diagnose GDM.

Working out if you have GDM – it all depends where you are! Sort of...

Say you attend an OGTT at a hospital using NICE criteria and get a result of a fasting blood glucose of 5.4mmol/L and a 2-hour result of 7.6mmol/L, then you will be told you do not have GDM. However, if your sister had the same results for the same tests but attended a hospital using the IADPSG/WHO criteria, she would be told she does have GDM because of the fasting blood glucose result of 5.4mmol/L.

Similarly if your sister in her IADPSG/WHO hospital had a FPG of 4.9mmol/L, a one-hour plasma glucose of 9.2mmol/L (remember, the IADPSG/WHO OGTT uses one-hour bloods as well) and a two-hour result of 8.3mmol/L, then she would be told she does not have GDM, but if she were attending your 'NICE' hospital, then she would be told she does have GDM (on account of her two-hour result being above 7.8mmol/L).

Now just in case you (or your hypothetical sister) have moved or are thinking of moving to the USA, you have a third set of OGTT diagnostic criteria to contend with. This is because the American College of Obstetricians and Gynaecologists (ACOG) have yet another set of results by which they diagnose GDM ($\geq$ 5.3mmol/L FPG, $\geq$ 10.0mmol/L at 1 hour, $\geq$ 8.6mmol/L at 2 hours and $\geq$7.8mol/L at 3 hours). And yes, the OGTT in units using these criteria does last THREE hours! Also in the USA 100g of glucose is given as opposed to the 75g elsewhere and the tests are done between 24 and 32 weeks gestation.

Meanwhile, the American Diabetes Association (ADA) have a different criterion and this is used in some UK maternity units. This criterion is TWO abnormal results out of the following: fasting >5.3mmol/L, 1-hour >10.0mmol/L and 2-hours >8.5mmol/L. The issue with this criterion is that women with high fasting but normal one-hour and two-hour results can be missed as far as diagnosis goes yet have pronounced GDM, because it is generally accepted that high fasting plasma glucose is more indicative of underlying glucose tolerance impairment than what happens following drinking loads of sugary drink.

It is even possible that the maternity unit you are attending for OGTT has its own criteria – **check with your midwife which set of criteria for GDM diagnosis are being used.**

Understanding the different criteria for being given a diagnosis of GDM and how they have been decided is a little complicated. However, it may help you decide how much (if any) intervention or treatment you want in the event that your OGTT result would have meant you were NOT given a GDM diagnosis had you undergone the OGTT elsewhere. This is a fairly common situation and one that AIMS comes across regularly. On the other hand, you may have been told you do not have GDM but nevertheless still want to be treated for GDM if you know you would have been diagnosed with it at a different hospital.

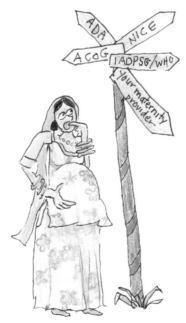

Odds Ratios (for readers who enjoy statistics)

The odds ratio (OR) is the odds of a particular outcome (for example, birth weight more than 4 kg or 8lbs 13oz) in a specific group (e.g. women with hyperglycaemia), compared to the odds of that same outcome occurring in a group with normal glucose levels (that is, the odds of a woman who does not have hyperglycaemia having a baby whose birth weight is more than 4kg or 8lbs 13oz).

If the Odds Ratio is 1 (OR = 1), then the outcome (high birth weight) is the same for both groups. There would be no difference in the numbers of babies weighing more than 4kg/8lbs 13oz born to women in either group. If the Odds Ratio is greater than 1 (OR >1), the outcome (high birth weight) is higher for the hyperglycaemic group and they would give birth to more babies weighing more than 4kg/8lbs 13oz than the women with normal glucose levels.

HAPO found that the Odds Ratio increased to 1.38 (OR = 1.38) for birth weight more than 4kg/8lbs 13oz for women whose fasting plasma glucose was 0.4mmol/L above the average (1 standard deviation for maths lovers). The average measurement for fasting plasma glucose was 4.5mmol/L.

This means that when a woman's fasting plasma glucose is elevated 0.4mmol/L from the average of 4.5mmol/L to 4.9mmol/L (still not high enough for a diagnosis of GDM by any of the current criteria), her baby is 0.38 or 38% more likely to have a birth weight more than 4kg/8lbs 13oz. For example, the overall rate of large babies weighing more than 4kg/8lbs 13oz is 1 in 10 births, but the OR of 1.38 would mean that on average, 138 large babies will be born to 1000 women with a fasting plasma glucose of 4.9mmol/L, as opposed to 100 large babies born to 1000 women with a fasting plasma glucose of 4.5mmol/L. Another way of putting this is that instead of the average 1 in 10 chance of a having a baby weighing more than 4kg/8lbs13oz, a woman with a fasting plasma glucose of 4.9mmol/L has just under a 1 in 7 chance of her baby weighing more than 4kg/8lbs 13oz.

Other HAPO Odds Ratios for 0.4mmol/L (or 1 standard deviation) above average fasting plasma glucose were:
1.55 for cord blood C-peptide above 90th percentile*
1.21 for pre-eclampsia
1.18 for shoulder dystocia or birth injury
1.11 for primary caesarean section (i.e. no previous CS)
1.08 for neonatal hypoglycaemia

Setting the diagnostic criteria for GDM at the level associated with these increases in odds ratios was rightly assessed by all the health organisations in Box 3 above as too low, and to lead to far too many women being diagnosed with GDM. However this illustration shows how some pregnancy outcomes (in this instance birth weight above 4kg/8lbs13oz) increase as maternal blood sugar levels increase.

The International Association of Diabetes and Pregnancy Study Groups and WHO have set their GDM plasma glucose diagnostic levels at those associated with an OR of 1.75 for **fetal macrosomia** and **hyperinsulinaemia**.

---

* C-peptide is a blood marker for high insulin levels over a period of time

Chapter 4:
Being diagnosed with GDM – what next?

Care and Treatment for GDM:
the first appointment

Once you have been diagnosed with GDM, you should be offered an appointment with a diabetes specialist midwife or nurse within a week, to discuss your blood results and to receive information about how to monitor your blood glucose levels and keep them as close to normal as you can.

This appointment is almost always in the maternity unit rather than the community. In fact, you may find that you do not see your community midwife again very much, if at all, as all your antenatal care may be offered at a specialist diabetes and pregnancy antenatal clinic at the hospital. If this is a problem for you, because of distance, travel or preference, tell the staff that you want to see your community midwife for as many antenatal appointments as possible. Many diabetes specialist midwives and nurses use phone and email contact to help you manage your GDM so that you do not have to go for hospital appointments all the time. In a few areas, such as Tower Hamlets in east London, women with GDM whose blood glucose levels remain within the target range through adjustments to diet and activity levels (discussed at length in this chapter) are offered care with community midwives rather than at a hospital clinic, with no increase in adverse outcomes (Sanghi, 2016).

You may want to take someone with you to these initial appointments as you will have lots of information to take in and questions to ask. Also, it will be helpful in the weeks to come if those close to you understand how and why you are trying to keep your blood glucose levels stable and as normal as you can. Try to write down or record questions on your phone as you think of them in the days between getting your results and your first appointment with the diabetes specialist midwife or nurse.

There are many social media forums for pregnant women, such as Netmums *www.netmums.com* or Baby Centre *www.babycentre.co.uk,* where you can ask other women questions or follow threads on topics such as GDM. This may help you to identify what you want to know or ask. Gestational Diabetes UK, *www.gestationaldiabetes. co.uk,* is a support group; their website has a lot of good nutritional advice, but some of the content is only available if you pay to join. It also has some good sections on induction of labour, homebirth, and waterbirth and a Facebook page with personal accounts and discussion. AIMS, *www.aims.org.uk,* and the Positive Birth Movement, *www.positivebirthmovement.org,* are also places to visit for help with choices and decisions. There is a short section signposting you to some key on-line resources towards the end of this book. Always remember that you can STILL make your own decisions on what care to accept, whether to stay with your community midwives for care or go to see the specialist ones, whether to follow the suggested food regime or not, whether to accept the medication offered or not, etc.

You will be offered self-monitoring of blood glucose, and dietary and lifestyle information. This is specifically designed to keep blood glucose levels as near normal as possible during pregnancy whilst making sure you have all the nutrition necessary for a healthy pregnancy.

You can also see a diabetes specialist dietitian who can explain and discuss how different foods affect blood glucose levels, and help you explore how they affect your personal glucose levels. The dietician will be able to suggest how to combine the different foods that you eat to better effect, and will help you make sense of food labels, portion sizes and so on. If you aren't offered an appointment with a diabetes specialist dietitian, you may want to ask for one as they have a great deal of knowledge and understanding of what, why and how we eat that might be very useful to you.

The dietitian can give you advice to help you reduce the amount of carbohydrate/sugars you eat by making adjustments to your diet, so that the amount of glucose your body is dealing with is more in line with the amount that the insulin you are producing can cope with. You will not be put on a slimming diet or be left feeling hungry or without enough to eat – the dietitian will give you lots of ideas on how to have enough good things to eat so that you are not hungry but you are eating less glucose-making food. Key to their guidance will be the replacement of foods with a **high glycaemic index (GI)** by foods with a **low glycaemic index**. There are many such lists and guides on the Internet, and two examples are given in the list of e-resources at the end of this book.

When you talk to the dietitian, try to be as accurate as you can about what you have been eating and the amounts, rather than tell them what you feel you should have been eating. You may also want to discuss any difficulties you are having in eating a better diet. This will make the discussion much more useful to you as their advice will be based on reality and not on a slightly idealised notion of your food intake. It may be useful to keep a food diary for a few days before you see the dietitian as this can be a good starting point for discussion – just note down when you eat, what you eat and the amounts you eat in a notebook, on the backs of envelopes, or on your phone. Or keep the wrappers or labels of food bought, such as sandwiches and crisps, ready-meals etc., as looking at these with the dietitian will help you to identify what you need to check on the labels. There are even apps available that let you scan food packet barcodes to record what you are eating.

Similarly, the advice you will be given about physical activity will be to help you, even when you are heavily pregnant, to use more energy, especially through muscle use. This will help you increase the rate at which your body uses the carbohydrate/sugars you do consume. Advice usually includes taking 30 to 60 minutes of exercise daily – walking, swimming, pregnancy exercise or yoga classes are good for most pregnant women – or going for a 30 minute walk after meals. Even a 10 to 15 minute walk immediately after a meal helps stabilise post-meal blood glucose levels and reduces them by up to 2mmols/L.

If you have persistent pelvic girdle pain, ask your midwife what physiotherapy support is available to you in your local NHS Trust to help you stay active. Borrow or buy a step counter or similar fitness aid, or download an app, or get a disused fitness monitor out of the drawer – these can be easy and useful ways of checking and increasing activity. Some of these have heart rate monitors and can also monitor how active you have been during the day.

A blood test called an HbA1c (pronounced H-B-A-one-C) will probably be offered at this stage – this is a way of assessing and monitoring average plasma glucose levels over the previous 4 to 6 weeks (8 to 12 weeks outside of pregnancy). Glucose joins onto the red blood cells or haemoglobin (Hb) in your blood and, as these cells are replaced about every 5 to 6 weeks (about 10 weeks outside of pregnancy), measuring the amount of glucose on them tells us how much glucose has been in your system, on average, during that period. If the result of the HbA1c test shows you have had high levels of glucose over the last weeks (above 48mmol/mol perhaps), then drug or insulin treatment may be offered.

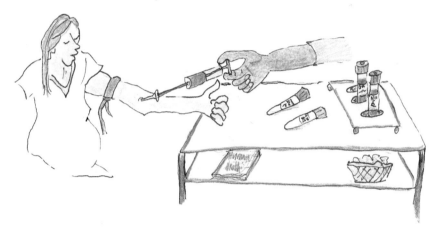

You will also be weighed because the dietitian will try to help you limit the amount of weight you gain in the last part of pregnancy. This is to avoid greater insulin resistance and consequent high plasma glucose levels, as discussed in Chapter 1, and to try to prevent your baby becoming too large. If you do gain more weight than advised, your dietitian will continue to help you find ways to eat well but limit your overall calorie intake.

You will be offered a blood glucose monitor, lancets for finger pricking, and strips for testing your blood glucose via the finger-tip pricks using the monitor. You will be shown how to use this and told how to get more stock when you run low. Make sure you are happy with how to use these before leaving. If you are needle-phobic or feel daunted by the idea of doing this, discuss this with the diabetes specialist midwife or nurse. They will be able to suggest how you might manage this. Most people do find the idea of self-glucose-monitoring daunting at first but nearly everyone manages it very well after a short time. This may be something you can get some tips and advice about via social media (see recommended sites earlier in this chapter and in the list of e-resources at the end of the book), or friends or relatives who have type 1 or type 2 diabetes.

You will also be given a blood glucose diary in which to record the results of your finger prick tests, usually first thing in the morning, before meals and one-hour after meals. If your blood glucose goes up, try to take stock of what you have eaten. Also try to note how exercise or stress affects your blood glucose levels. Some people, for example, find that fruit or fruit juice raises their glucose levels, others that fried food does this. Try to follow the dietary advice you have been given as this is designed to maintain stable glucose levels throughout the 24-hours of the day to ensure that your and your baby's cells have adequate but not harmful levels of glucose. The results of the finger prick tests will enable you to identify what does and doesn't suit your body in terms of glucose levels. You will be given targets for your blood glucose results, such as:

≥5.3mmol/L for fasting glucose;
≥7.4mmol/L for 1 hour after a meal (called 'post-prandial');
≥6.7mmol/L for 2 hours after a meal.

The targets you are given may differ depending on your BMI. For example, you may be given fasting and one-hour post-meal targets of 5.3mmol and 7.8mmol if your BMI was below 30 at booking, but be given 5.3mmol and 7.0mmol targets if your BMI was above 30 at booking, as your baby is more likely to become large if you have a high BMI.

Lifestyle and dietary changes usually work best if those around you at home also follow them. Discuss this with your partner and family. If you are switching to granary bread, more vegetables and protein, and brown basmati rice, for example, it will be easier if your family make the same changes, not only in terms of shopping and food preparation but also in terms of sustaining the change.

Many women cannot tolerate sugary breakfast cereals and even those that are promoted as healthier versions often have a high GI index. One or two slices of granary bread with some protein such as eggs, peanut butter or cheese is a much better breakfast in terms of morning blood glucose levels and a good alternative to breakfast cereals.

If your fasting glucose result was high (above 7mmol/L) you are likely to be offered insulin with or without the addition of metformin even at this early stage (see later in this chapter for discussion of these drug therapies). Drug therapy is always a supplement to and not a replacement for lifestyle interventions in GDM – the latter will also be very important later on as I will discuss in Chapter 6. If your fasting plasma glucose is between 6 and 6.9mmol/L, you may be offered insulin if your baby is already showing signs of being large or has a lot of amniotic fluid around him or her.

[NB judging a baby's weight in the womb is not always accurate and scans tend to become less accurate in later pregnancy (Mackenzie *et al.*, 2016). Amniotic fluid measurement is not totally accurate either, and measurements on the high side do not always indicate a problem.

See *https://midwifethinking.com/2013/08/14/amniotic-fluid-volume-too-much-too-little-or-who-knows* for further information on the latter.]

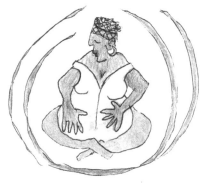

Importantly, you will be provided with contact telephone numbers so you can seek advice, support and information at any time. Diabetes teams use email and telephone contact a great deal to stay in touch with their clients, and will want you to tell them if you have any concerns as soon as possible, so contact them if you have any worries or queries. It is particularly important, for example, that you contact the team if your plasma glucose readings are very high or you become unwell, as either of these may indicate a need to change treatment. Your diabetes team will give you guidance on this.

Care and Treatment for GDM: the second appointment

Normally you will be offered a second appointment a week after the first appointment to discuss your blood glucose diary, how you are getting on, and what to do next in some depth. This appointment will be with the specialist diabetes and pregnancy team and will likely include seeing a diabetologist (a specialist diabetes doctor), perhaps an obstetrician as well, and/or the specialist diabetes midwife or dietitian at the same appointment, depending on your individual situation. This is when all the information you have collected in your blood glucose diary will be looked at with you, and a course of treatment or other action is discussed with you; you then have the information you need to decide what action you wish to take, if any.

Ongoing care and interventions, including treatment with metformin or insulin

Following a diagnosis of GDM, you will be offered antenatal appointments with the specialist team quite frequently – weekly to four-weekly, depending on your condition. One of the things that women with GDM often find helpful and supportive is being looked after by a small team and seeing the same people during pregnancy and, to a lesser extent, after giving birth. You will usually be seen by the same people and be able to build up a relationship with them over a number of appointments. You should also have contact numbers and/or email addresses to ask for information and support between appointments.

Two interventions that you will be offered are additional ultrasound scans and umbilical artery doppler measurement (this is a technique to assess blood flow between you and your baby)[10]. These will be scheduled for around 32 and 36 weeks and their purpose is to assess your baby's growth and other markers of well-being, such as the amount of amniotic fluid and the blood flow through the umbilical cord. If you are diagnosed with GDM before 28 weeks, you will be offered a scan to assess fetal growth and the amount of amniotic fluid at 28 weeks (NICE, 2015).

When you get a diagnosis of GDM it means that you will normally be expected to have your baby on the obstetric unit in the hospital. However, you are the person who decides where to give birth, and

---

10 See AIMS book *Ultrasound? Unsound* for information about safety issues relating to ultrasound in pregnancy.

the hospital trust's guidelines are not something you need to follow. If you would like to have your baby at home, this is entirely your decision and the hospital trust must support you. It is quite likely that the trust will not permit you to birth your baby on the midwife-led unit, if they have one, and they do have the right to decide this. However, it is important to remember that for women whose blood glucose levels have been well maintained, and whose babies do not appear to be overly large, it is likely that there are no additional risks when compared to a woman who has not developed GDM. In that case, it may be possible to negotiate access to a midwife-led unit if you would like to birth there. You can make an appointment with a consultant or a senior midwife to talk over the options for care and how your plans and needs might be met by the maternity service.

Whilst you will be offered a revised package of care after being diagnosed with GDM, with the expectation that this is acceptable to you, it cannot be imposed on you and there is always room for discussion and adaptation – consent must be given by you, not coerced from you, and you must be in agreement with any plans for your care, not have them made for you by others. Most doctors and midwives will try to suggest alternatives if you are not happy with the usual package of care. Indeed the NICE 2015 Guideline on Diabetes in Pregnancy states:

*Tailor blood glucose-lowering therapy to the blood glucose and **personal preferences of the woman with gestational diabetes**.* (NICE, 2015, p.19, my emphasis)

If your GDM is well-controlled by diet and exercise, and you do not go into labour before 40 weeks, then you will be offered a further ultrasound scan at 40 weeks' gestation. You are likely to come under some pressure to agree to induction of labour[11] as you reach 38 to 40 weeks unless your GDM is well-controlled by lifestyle measures (induction of labour and making decisions about induction is discussed a little later in this chapter).

Many women do maintain plasma glucose within the target range through lifestyle change and monitoring as discussed in the previous section. But around a third to half of women do need medication to maintain plasma glucose in the range associated with fewer problems for mother and baby (see Box 4 on page 64). So, if you are one of those women who continues to have high plasma glucose readings despite the lifestyle changes you make, you will have to assess the risks associated with the high readings and decide what to do – continue in the same way or try drug therapy to reduce plasma glucose – with either metformin (a tablet), insulin (an injection), or both.

A **systematic review** of treatment for GDM found that treatment (insulin, oral medication, lifestyle changes, blood glucose monitoring alone or in any combination), compared with no treatment, was associated with decreases in incidence of pre-eclampsia (by 35%) and large baby (by 50%), but that induction rates increased by 33% (Alwan et al., 2009). They also looked at death or injury to the baby. Although there were not any statistically significant differences in any single severe adverse outcome (they are too rare to assess statistically in isolation), when they combined these adverse outcomes (shoulder dystocia, nerve palsy, fracture to arm or shoulder bone, death during labour or in the first week), there was a 68% decrease in the treatment group, though the absolute risk remains low.

---

11 See AIMS book *Inducing Labour: Making Informed Decisions*

However, the authors concluded that, whilst treatment of GDM was beneficial, there was no clear evidence on whether dietary and lifestyle advice or more intensive interventions, such as medication or insulin, were more effective at preventing complications (Alwan et al., 2009). This applies even to mild levels of GDM with blood sugar levels just above the threshold for GDM diagnosis (Landon et al., 2009).

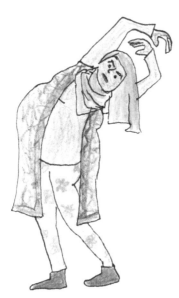

Whilst treatment reduces the likelihood of the adverse outcomes above, it does not do away with them entirely – you may still develop pre-eclampsia or experience shoulder dystocia, as will some women without GDM – nor does having untreated GDM mean that you will necessarily have any of these problems. What it does mean is that treatment will reduce the likelihood of them happening.

I will briefly outline the main treatments offered in addition to lifestyle changes below, and add a little more about the sort of care you are likely to be offered. It is up to you to decide what to accept – even with a diagnosis of GDM you still have the right to decide: to consider the information you are given, and to weigh up the benefits, risks and the alternatives, and to consider how you want to proceed as an individual, a couple and a family. Some of the pressure on you will be time-related: you are often asked to make decisions at an appointment or from week to week. If you need more time at any stage, don't be afraid to say so; state that you need more time to think it over and discuss it with someone else, whether it be an hour, a day or a week depending on the situation. A useful sentence from veteran midwife Mary Cronk is, "Thank you very much for your advice. I will consider what you have said and let you know my decision".

The BRAIN approach to health decisions

You may find BRAIN a helpful acronym during appointment visits. BRAIN[12] stands for BENEFITS, RISKS, ALTERNATIVES, INTUITION and NOTHING and many people have found it a good way to discuss and think about health decisions with health professionals and together as a family or couple.

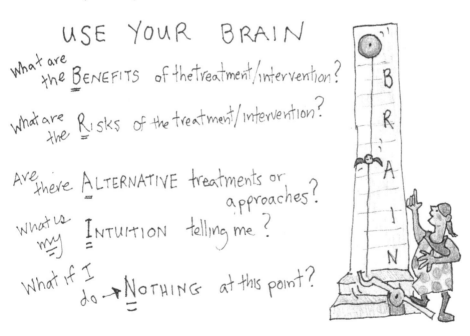

USE YOUR BRAIN

What are the BENEFITS of the treatment/intervention?

What are the RISKS of the treatment/intervention?

Are there ALTERNATIVE treatments or approaches?

What is my INTUITION telling me?

What if I do → NOTHING at this point?

---

12 BRAIN (formerly BRAN) has been widely quoted and used as a medical decision-making tool for several decades, I have been unable to trace its origin.

Most maternity units have small specialist teams consisting of an obstetrician with a special interest in diabetes, a consultant diabetologist with a special interest in pregnancy, and specialist dietitians, nurses and midwives who hold dedicated antenatal clinics for women with diabetes and GDM. Health professionals like diabetologists working mainly with ill people are accustomed to their patients accepting the treatment they offer and may be taken aback if you, who are not ill, do not readily agree to it. However, recognising that this is what they may be used to, rather than a lack of interest or willingness to discuss options with you, may help you ask questions or make suggestions.

If, at any stage after you have been diagnosed with GDM, your blood glucose exceeds the targets you have been given on a number of occasions (usually three or more during a week), you will be advised to start medication.

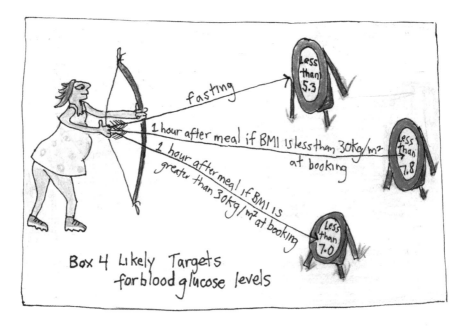

Box 4 Likely Targets for blood glucose levels

Medication for GDM

Metformin

Metformin is the most common drug used to treat type 2 diabetes and it is also used to treat GDM. Metformin is offered when plasma glucose levels remain high despite lifestyle change, or are very high on first diagnosis of GDM. For many people, it has been found to be as effective as insulin in controlling plasma glucose levels (Lindsay, 2012). It acts by:

*   making the insulin you produce more efficient at transporting glucose from your blood into your cells;
*   reducing the amount of pre-glucose (called glycogen) made in the liver;
*   increasing the amount of glucose used by muscle and fat cells;
*   reducing the amount of glucose absorbed by the intestine.

All of which helps to lower plasma glucose levels. Metformin has been found to be as effective as a 15 to 20 minute walk, which reinforces the importance of physical activity as the first line of treatment (with dietary changes). If you do not want to take metformin, additional exercise and particularly more daily walking may help reduce your blood glucose levels. The dose is normally initially 500mg (1 tablet) daily but is commonly increased to 1500mg daily as pregnancy progresses.

Metformin cannot cause maternal hypoglycaemia (low blood sugar). It is often used to treat polycystic ovary syndrome as well as type 2 diabetes, so there is quite a lot known about it in relation to pregnancy and breastfeeding.

The main side effect of metformin is gastro-intestinal upset in the form of nausea, vomiting, stomach upset or diarrhoea which occur in about

I in 5 people taking it. Side effects can be minimised by starting on a low dose and building the dose up gradually, increasing the dose by one tablet every 3 – 4 days ("Start Low, Go Slow!"); also by taking the tablet immediately before or with food. Around I in 50 women have to discontinue metformin because of gastro-intestinal side-effects and around I in 10 have to reduce the dose, but over three-quarters of women report satisfaction with metformin (Lindsay, 2012).

Metformin is also associated with reduced weight gain during pregnancy by an average of about 1.5kg, and avoiding excessive weight gain is known to improve pregnancy outcomes (Rowan, 2008).

Metformin crosses the placenta and research so far has not shown any problems for babies, including longer-term metabolic disorder in children exposed to it whilst in the womb *after* the first 13 weeks of pregnancy up to the age of 7 to 9 years (Rowan *et al.*, 2011). The following paragraphs outline the research which is being undertaken at the time of writing (2017) and there is likely to be more research, so I recommend that you ask your doctor or midwife about this as information may become available over the next few years.

Children whose mothers were treated with metformin or insulin for GDM are currently being followed up closely over a number of years in Australia and New Zealand. Those children whose mothers took metformin show a slightly more favourable fat distribution at 2 years of age (less fat in the abdomen and around organs such as the liver and heart), which may lead to greater insulin sensitivity and less diabetes over the longer term though this is not confirmed (Rowan *et al.*, 2011). However, a recent review of metformin use in pregnancy advised caution and the need for more research data, particularly on the effects on male reproductive organs (Bertoldo *et al.*, 2014).

Metformin also appears in breast milk at about 0.65% of the maternal dose. Because women with polycystic ovarian syndrome (PCOS) or type 2 diabetes often take it throughout pregnancy and during breastfeeding, there have been some longer-term studies of babies exposed to metformin through breastmilk, but no adverse effects have been found (Feig, 2012). Because all treatment for GDM stops at birth, the amount of metformin that a baby born to someone who had been taking it during pregnancy for GDM would be exposed to would be a lot less than that which babies of women with type 2 diabetes or PCOS are exposed to.

The official pharmacological advice (The British National Formulary) is that metformin appears to be safe in breastfeeding but caution is advised in relation to breastfeeding premature babies or those with renal problems.

Metformin can also be used in addition to insulin injections (see below) so that the amount of insulin needed is less. This is because metformin makes both the insulin given by injection, and that made by your pancreas, work more efficiently. Around half of all women initially treated with metformin also need insulin by the end of pregnancy (Rowan et al., 2008). If you prefer not to take metformin you can request insulin instead.

Insulin

Insulin is a hormone produced in the pancreas that enables your body cells to use glucose for energy. It is essential to all mammalian life. Modern insulin for injection is much more sophisticated and better used by the human body than that of 30 years ago. Today we mostly use synthetic insulins (insulin analogues) rather than animal-derived insulin.

Nearly half of women with GDM who are treated with metformin also require insulin to maintain plasma glucose in the advised range (Box 4). Many women choose to use insulin instead of metformin because its glucose-lowering effects are faster, it has fewer side-effects, and it does not cross the placenta. So do not think that you need to try metformin first; you may prefer to use insulin as it does have these advantages over metformin.

You may have a short-acting insulin at one meal time, or every meal time, and some women also need a longer-acting insulin through the day, between meals or through the night. It will depend on your individual plasma glucose picture as kept by you in your diary.

Insulin comes in easy-to-use injection 'pens' with short needles and is self-administered into the fat of your upper arm or thigh once to five times a day – the maximum schedule is short-acting insulin immediately before each meal three times a day and a longer acting insulin that acts over 12-24 hours once or twice a day. Most women find it much less painful than the finger pricks they are already doing.

You will be given lots of help and information about how to take the insulin and a 24-hour telephone support number if you are prescribed insulin. It sounds more daunting than it is – try to talk to someone with experience of self-administering insulin, either in person or via social media, for their insights and advice. If you really cannot bear the idea, then do talk to your midwife or doctor at the diabetes antenatal clinic, using the BRAIN approach outlined on page 63. Ask for time to consider the matter if you feel that would help – taking a day or two to explore the matter further is perfectly reasonable.

As well as injection pens of insulin, you will also be given alcohol wipes, a sharps bin for the safe disposal of needles, and information on how to recognise and treat hypoglycaemia. Hypoglycaemia is when your blood sugar goes very low because of having more insulin in your system than you need, either because you have given yourself too much, or you have delayed eating after giving yourself the insulin injection, or you are ill, or have done a lot of exercise – basically you have not taken in enough carbohydrates to use up the extra insulin you have injected.

Hypoglycaemia

The signs of hypoglycaemia are:
* Tingling in mouth, tongue or fingers
* Blurred or double vision
* Increased sweating
* Heart beating fast
* Feeling agitated or behaving oddly
* Sudden poor concentration
* Slurred speech

Treatment is by quickly eating or drinking something with enough sugar to use up the insulin causing the problem. One of the following is best:

* 4 jelly babies
* A glass of orange juice or non-diet fizzy drink
* 5 glucose or dextrose tablets
* A prepared glucose drink prescribed for hypoglycaemia by your doctor

You will also be given information about safe driving when using insulin – the common reminder is "Five before you Drive" – i.e. your blood glucose should be tested and be 5mmol/L or more before you drive, to minimise the possibility of a hypoglycaemic event, and needs to be checked every two hours.

Glibenclamide

On rare occasions Glibenclamide[13] is used for the treatment of GDM. It might be offered to you as an alternative to metformin if side-effects are a problem, or in addition to metformin if plasma glucose remains high on metformin alone and you decline insulin. Balsells *et al.* (2015) showed in their review of the use of glibenclamide, metformin and insulin for the treament of GDM that glibenclamide is the least-preferred treatment option. It crosses the placenta and is associated with higher rates of neonatal hypoglycaemia (discussed in Chapter 5), and **macrosomia**.

There is limited information about use of the drug in breastfeeding but it has not been detected in breastmilk, and no adverse effects have been detected. As it would be stopped as soon as the baby is born in the case of GDM, there is no reason not to breastfeed if you have been taking glibenclamide during pregnancy for GDM.

If you are admitted to hospital during pregnancy

Make sure you or a health care professional continues to monitor your blood glucose before breakfast and one hour after all meals.

---

13 Glibenclamide belongs to a group of drugs known as sulphonylureas. Others include glipizide, and gliclazide. Sulphonylureas are teratogenic (can cause fetal abnormalities) and should not be taken around the time of conception or in the first 12 weeks of pregnancy.

Make sure the diabetes team know you have been admitted. You may have been admitted for something that has nothing to do with your GDM, but someone from the specialist team will make sure that you and the ward staff have a plan to help you manage your GDM as well as you can.

If you are admitted to hospital for more than 24 hours for any reason when you have GDM, you should be seen by a dietitian to discuss your dietary needs as the routine hospital food menu you are offered may not be the best for keeping your plasma glucose levels stable. The dietitian will help you order the food you need to keep your glucose levels within your target range. If a dietitian does not come to see you on your second day, you may want to ask to see one.

Induction of labour

If your GDM is controlled by diet alone and your baby is thought to be growing at a normal rate and to have a normal amount of amniotic fluid (the water surrounding your baby in the womb) at a 36 week scan (if you decide to have this) or appointment, induction of labour may be discussed at your later appointments. If you have any complications on top of or as a result of your GDM, it will probably be discussed earlier than this and you may be advised to have your labour induced. It is important to remember that elective caesarean section is an alternative to induction and that this needs to be included in any discussion. Whilst surgery should never be offered or accepted without good reason, exploring all options is important and caesarean section can be the best option in some situations.

In uncomplicated GDM pregnancies, induction of labour by 40 weeks and 6 days is advised by NICE because of a small increased risk of having a stillborn baby (NICE, 2015). There is no indication for induction before this if your GDM is diet-controlled and your baby has a normal growth pattern.

There is a very small increased risk of stillbirth in GDM, which is probably greater the higher your plasma glucose is. No-one really understands why some babies die at this late stage of pregnancy, or why this happens more often with GDM. Whilst high glucose levels increase the risk, a small number of babies do die when glucose levels are not so high. There is no glucose level at which anyone can say that the risk doesn't exist, though it is very small for women with GDM which is well-controlled by lifestyle measures (diet and physical activity). It is important to remember that the stillbirth rate is very low for women with and without GDM. For example, at 40 weeks gestation in women without GDM approximately 1 baby in 2300 births is stillborn. For women with GDM at the same gestation it is approximately 1 baby in 1800 births (Rosenstein et al., 2012). At 42 weeks, the rates are approximately 1 in 1100 and 1 in 870 respectively. So with GDM the risk increases but is still low, especially where blood sugars are well-controlled.

To explore the level of risk more, let's look at the large study done in the USA by Rosenstein and colleagues. They attempted to assess the level of risk of stillbirth in a highly diverse and multi-ethnic Californian population by looking at nearly 200,000 GDM pregnancies and comparing the outcomes with almost 4 million pregnancies without GDM in the same period. Their study found that there was no benefit to intervening through induction of labour in an otherwise uncomplicated GDM pregnancy before 39 weeks as far as any risk of mortality is concerned, and the benefits thereafter were very small. They estimated that at 39 weeks gestation, 1500 women would have to be induced to prevent one baby dying and at 40 weeks 1300 women would have to be induced to prevent one baby dying (Rosenstein *et al.*, 2012). As induction of labour itself has a number of disadvantages and risks, NICE has concluded that the costs (physical, emotional and financial to women, babies and the health service) outweigh the benefits, and that other approaches such as careful monitoring and treatment are preferable up to at least 40 weeks and 6 days.

The other reason commonly given for the induction of labour is **macrosomia** or large baby (over 4kg or 8lbs 13oz), where it is thought that an earlier birth will prevent the baby growing to the extent that his or her shoulders prove difficult to birth (**shoulder dystocia**). Difficulty freeing the baby's shoulder from the front of the pelvis (symphysis pubis) can occasionally result in injury to the baby's shoulder or arm, such as a palsy or a fracture, or sometimes an episiotomy or tear to the mother's vaginal wall or, in rare instances, to brain injury or death.

Shoulder dystocia can be frightening for the parents as it is treated as an emergency with people often flying into the room in response to an emergency alarm being pressed. The treatment is actually fairly straightforward and well-rehearsed by all maternity staff: the mother's legs are supported and held outwards and pressure from the ball of an attendant's hand applied above the symphysis pubis to free the baby's shoulder through a rocking movement AND/OR mother being helped onto all-fours and the posterior shoulder being born first, with the stuck anterior shoulder following after. (This can be done in any order but is usually done in the order given here as shoulder dystocia appears to be less common when women are on all-fours in the first place.) The few minutes this takes and the sudden appearance of unknown staff can sometimes be traumatic, but your midwife should explain quickly and calmly what is happening and how you can complete the birthing of your baby. Most babies are born quickly and safely by these manoeuvres.

However, induction of labour for babies thought to be large is controversial. First, fetal weight can only be estimated and, even using ultrasound, estimates can often be inaccurate. Secondly, many women birth large babies without any problems. Thirdly, most cases of shoulder dystocia occur in average-sized babies (though proportionally more in larger babies). And finally, we know that being upright and mobile is less likely to result in problems giving birth. Unfortunately, induction of labour means you are more likely to be semi-supine and confined to a bed, unless you plan for and get help and support in maintaining upright and active positions during labour.

Although induction for big babies has been shown to reduce shoulder dystocia from 68/1000 births to 41/1000 births and fractures of the babies' collarbones from 20/1000 births to 4/1000 births compared with waiting for labour to begin, there is no difference in rates of nerve injury to babies' upper arms, or the health of babies at birth as measured by Apgar scores or cord blood pH (Cochrane infographic 'Induction of labour for big babies' 2016). NICE, the body that sets standards for health care, has concluded:

In the absence of any other indications, induction of labour should not be carried out simply because a healthcare professional suspects a baby is large for gestational age (macrosomic). (NICE, 2008)

Likewise, the Royal College of Obstetricians and Gynaecologists (RCOG) do not recommend either induction of labour or caesarean section for the prevention of shoulder dystocia in larger babies as neither can be shown to improve outcomes (RCOG, 2013).

One of the reasons you may be offered induction of labour in some units is if your baby's growth accelerates, particularly between 32 and 36 weeks. This may be due to high blood glucose levels or not enough treatment of your GDM, and may mean that your baby is laying down extra fat deposits around his or her shoulders and abdomen. In this instance, you may be asked to consider induction after 38 weeks. Make sure you understand exactly what the situation is – how big is the baby estimated to be? What are the chances of successful induction at this stage of pregnancy? Have you given birth to large babies before? Are there increased risks? Are there other treatment options?

The decision to accept or decline induction of labour, at any gestation and regardless of whether your pregnancy is complicated or not, will be a personal one, depending on and weighing up the various adverse elements of induced labour against the small increase in the risk of perinatal death or some of the problems associated with having a larger baby. Induction of labour is discussed fully in the AIMS book *Inducing Labour: Making Informed Decisions* by Sara Wickham, which is also available as an e-book, but the main advantages and disadvantages are summarised in Box 5 overleaf.

Box 5 Some advantages/disadvantages of INDUCTION of LABOUR

ADVANTAGES	DISADVANTAGES
• Reduces the small risk of perinatal death after 39 weeks • Increases certainty about period of baby's arrival	• Requires hospitalisation or longer hospitalisation • More vaginal exams • More time on a bed • Artificial rupture of membranes • Sharper labour contractions/surges • Likely to mean an IV drip • More continuous fetal heart monitoring required • More likely to have pharmacological pain relief (drugs) or an epidural • More likely to give birth by Caesarean Section or forceps/Ventouse • Increased liklihood of fetal distress • Increased rate of shoulder dystocia

Many women find it really helps to consider this issue and read about it early, as it is likely to come up in later discussions with your healthcare team even if there is no mention at your first couple of appointments. You can use the BRAIN approach outlined earlier in this chapter and summarised below, use social media to find out how other women have reached decisions, and visit the AIMS website. Induction of labour is a big decision, whether accepted or declined, so be honest about your concerns and trust your intuition about what is right for you and your baby. Your decision, for or against induction, will be a good one and right for you, if you come to it freely as a woman, a mother, and a partner.

The BRAIN approach to considering induction of labour:

* What are the <u>benefits</u> of induction of labour for me/my baby/ at this time?
* What are the <u>risks</u> of induction of labour for me/my baby/at this time?
* Are there <u>alternative</u> approaches to induction or for continuing with my pregnancy, taking my GDM into account?
* What is my <u>intuition</u> telling me?
* What if I do <u>nothing</u> at this point?

Blood glucose monitoring and control during labour

You or (if you are unable to do so, such as during a caesarean section) one of the health professionals caring for you will continue to monitor your blood glucose during labour if you are on any glucose-lowering medication that may cause hypoglycaemia (usually insulin). Your blood glucose should remain between 4 and 7mmol/L during labour to minimise the risk of hypoglycaemia in your baby after birth (see next chapter). Depending on how you are managing your GDM, a plan for doing so during labour should be made with you by the diabetes specialist midwife or someone else in the specialist team during your later antenatal visits. Make sure you are clear and in agreement about that plan and what you will need to do or have with you in terms of equipment and medication.

Apart from the points that have been discussed above, your GDM is unlikely to affect the course of your labour or the care you receive. You should be able to move freely, use a birth pool and make choices in the same way as any woman without GDM. You may wish to discuss your birth plan with your diabetes specialist team to ensure that your choices are noted and understood before you go into labour.

Women's Experiences

I received a short letter informing me I had gestational diabetes one Saturday morning when I was about 29 weeks pregnant. I remember it clearly because I was due to meet some friends for lunch that day and it threw me into a panic because I was worried about what I should eat. And over the week that followed, I read too many online forums and articles about gestational diabetes until I finally collapsed in tears wailing to my husband that I'd damaged our unborn baby by eating too many sweets! Up until then, I'd had a straightforward and happy pregnancy. I was fit and healthy; I am a runner and had continued to run several times a week until about week 22 of pregnancy when it became too difficult. **Sophie, GDM with first baby**

I attended a group session with other mums who had GDM, to receive information about healthy eating, how to manage blood sugar through diet and exercise, and also to be given our blood sugar testing kits and to be shown how to use them 4 times a day – once as soon as you wake and once one hour after each main meal. This group meeting, although lovely to meet other mums going through the same thing, was a little like what I imagine going to an AA meeting would be like! It was a little surreal, and I certainly felt a little anxious about it and almost as though I had done something wrong in order to be diagnosed with GDM. I wanted to shout out that I eat healthily and do mummy fitness classes and run around after a 4 year old all day! **Stacey, GDM with second baby**

The first meeting with the GDM nurse was great. I made sure I asked her for a list of what I could eat to get me started, and got it written down before I left. At the time, I was driving fair distances for work and was concerned about maintaining my levels. I really feel that food diaries and snacks would've helped a lot. I joined a Facebook page a friend suggested and found this the best support I could have wished for. I managed to control my GDM solely by diet and was delighted that I avoided meds. I had one day of spikes leading into a weekend so I phoned the GDM team on a Friday afternoon who made me a provisional appointment for the Saturday in case things hadn't settled. They were back to normal the following morning! It was helpful to make people at work aware, as it meant us all getting into good habits and a proper lunch rather than just grabbing something quickly from a garage forecourt! **Nicola, GDM with first baby**

I was lucky enough to be able to control my diabetes with my diet. I found that what I could eat was very specific to me and that some of the things that were suggested made my levels high. My husband even had to bring food to me in hospital as what was offered was not suitable for me. I had a kit and tested my levels before and after every meal, first thing in the morning and last thing at night. I found that it was a bit 'trial and error' and eventually concluded that I always needed lots of protein in my meals to balance out any carbohydrates or fruit, and I totally gave up refined sugar. I have never felt so good! *Joanna, GDM with second baby*

After a week or so of testing it became clear that it was my morning levels that resulted in some higher results after breakfast (a healthy breakfast of refined sugar-free homemade muesli with natural yogurt and berries), so I had to play around with different breakfasts to work out what would bring that reading in under the required level. That turned out to be 2 slices of low GI granary toast with almond butter, which I stuck to for the rest of my pregnancy! *Stacey, GDM with second baby*

It was first suspected that I may have gestational diabetes when a very observant midwife detected 4++++ of glucose in my urine at a routine antenatal appointment. She sent me for an OGTT and I was diagnosed the next day. The following few days were a whirlwind of appointments with consultants, diabetic nurses and dietitians, and initially I was trying to control the diabetes with diet. After a couple of weeks however it became clear that it was getting worse despite the fact that I was watching what I was eating, and I was put onto insulin. Although I was terrified at the prospect of injections, the reality was that the finger pricks were more painful than the injections – if you got the right spot you actually didn't feel them!! It took a few weeks for the diabetes to stabilise and even then I had to crank up the amount of insulin I was taking quite quickly. I had a couple of hypos which were not pleasant at all. *Nicki, GDM with first baby*

I have nothing but positive vibes to send anyone with GDM. To be regularly checked, get an extra scan and have a team of specialists to contact (other than my midwife) was amazing and I felt so reassured and relaxed. And the other thing... it's more common than you first realise and really isn't all doom and gloom. *Nicola, GDM with first baby*

I had to ring up for the results later the same day and was told that I had GDM. I was given no further useful information in this phone call, just told to come to a clinic a week later. I found this very stressful. I was upset about finding I had GDM, I didn't know what it meant for the baby or me and I wanted to start doing something about it immediately. Having to wait a week for more information was not good for me. I went out and bought some books on diabetes which had small amounts of information on GDM, but at least they helped me to start trying to eat the right things.

I went to the clinic at the hospital the following week and saw a midwife, a consultant, a dietician and maybe others, it was quite a conveyor belt of appointments. I was given and shown how to use a blood sugar monitoring kit, which was fine, and told about what levels I should try to keep my sugars between. I wasn't very impressed with the dietary advice – I was given a leaflet which said things like have a rich tea biscuit instead of a digestive, whereas everything I had read lead me to think I shouldn't be eating any biscuits at all. I didn't particularly follow their advice but instead followed a strict low GI diet while still ensuring that I was eating sufficient protein, calcium, fat and vitamins/minerals. I measured my blood sugar 4 times per day, which I quickly got used to and was very successful at keeping within the limits they had given me, so much so that I lost weight and was lighter by the end of my pregnancy than I had been at my booking appointment. *Rebecca, GDM with second baby*

I was quickly seen by a consultant and nutritionalist and well supported to successfully manage to control my sugar levels by diet alone, by eating little and often the foods discussed with me by the nutritionist. **Soshanna, GDM with third baby**

The 4 times a day testing, together with the regular appointments in the hospital were extremely time consuming and also difficult to fit in, given that I was working part time and I have a 4 year old too, and without family nearby. Going to the hospital always tended to raise my blood pressure too - they are not my favourite places, hence the wish to have a home birth. I felt that given my consistently good readings and the baby scans being good, that it was a little unnecessary to have to go to the hospital so regularly. We wondered whether perhaps, where a pregnant lady is maintaining good blood sugar levels and health, this can be monitored through routine midwife appointments. **Stacey, GDM with second baby**

I found myself sucked into a system and there didn't seem to be any way out. My first of many hospital appointments involved going into about four different rooms at our local hospital seeing various people, none of whom introduced themselves or gave me any coherent answers to my questions. It transpired my blood sugar at my glucose tolerance test had only been 0.1 above the recommended levels but this was never mentioned again. It was irrelevant it appeared. I had Gestational Diabetes and therefore I must follow that care pathway. I was given a blood sugar monitoring kit and told to test my blood four times a day for the rest of my pregnancy. I fully intended to do everything I was told by the professionals to make sure my baby was safe. I took notes at my appointments and was determined not to go onto medication so I followed everything I was told by the nutritionist I saw to the letter. In some ways, it was actually pretty easy and the advice straightforward. I just needed not to go overboard on high sugar snacks, and space all my food out throughout the day so as not to spike my sugar levels. What I found most difficult, was that my antenatal care was transferred to a hospital consultant, actually a number of consultants, as over the months that followed I saw different ones. I don't remember seeing a midwife to talk to again, except for the myriad of ones who came to measure my bump at my bi-weekly hospital appointments to check my baby was not growing too big. **Rebecca, GDM with second baby**

I could keep my blood sugar under targets pretty easily by following a low carbohydrate diet. Until this point I was booked in with the homebirth team. They kicked me off immediately and I was suddenly at an appointment with an awful consultant who was telling me I would be induced at 40 weeks or I was risking my baby being stillborn (underlined in my notes!!). I was devastated about the way I was treated. I asked her for her evidence to back up this plan of action and she couldn't provide it. I critiqued all the research I could find and found no evidence to support the fact that I should be induced at 40 weeks as per her plan. I decided to move to another local hospital. They were much better, and I met with the supervisor of midwives and we agreed I could use the birth centre up until 42 weeks (hospital policy is to induce at 41+5 even for low risk pregnancies). I was happy with that plan. If I had more support I may have pushed for a homebirth but I did have some concerns about the fact I was diagnosed quite late, and I felt the birth centre was an ok compromise given the circumstances. They then started putting a lot of pressure on to be induced by 41 weeks. I was so stressed out. I limped on feeling totally unsupported until 42 weeks and then I knew my chance to use the birth centre was gone. So I was induced, and it was a difficult birth. My son was born happy and healthy though, 8lbs 1oz. We had a tough first year though and I am sure the birth contributed to that. **Lisa, GDM with first baby**

The hospital said they would give me a call the next day if it showed as positive. I had a voice message on my mobile the next day and my heart sank. I then knew before speaking to anybody that I had GDM. At this point I didn't realise the impact it would have on me over the next coming weeks. I was booked into the diabetic clinic. I turned up with a group of other women in similar situations and was given a kit with a glucose monitor to test first thing in the morning and after every meal. All the other women in the room had already had GDM in a previous pregnancy. It was all new to me. They quickly ran through diet and what you could eat or alternatives to what you were already eating. I was enjoying my pregnancy until this point.

I don't particularly like needles, so doing the finger pricking test was a bit of an issue for me until I got used to it. I sat in this room with my hands sweating the first time I had to do the prick test. The diabetic nurse did it for me as I was scared to do it, and it wasn't as bad as I expected and got easier the more I pricked! Sometimes it really hurt my finger depending on where I pricked. It was annoying having to carry the kit around and remembering an hour after each meal to do it. I was shocked by some of the things that I ate which pushed my blood sugar levels really high for example: cereals. I tried all sorts and the ones that I thought would not be high, such as porridge and Weetabix, still pushed my levels higher than the 7.8 I was aiming for. I had been enjoying pregnancy because I thought this is the first time in many years I don't have to think about watching my weight or dieting because it was inevitable that I would gain weight. Once diagnosed with GDM this was completely taken away and, as always in life, I had to watch again what I was eating and drinking every meal. Some days especially near the end of pregnancy I was so tired I had some chocolate or something sweet to boost my energy. Afterwards, I felt guilty and worried I may harm my baby. I also worried that my baby was growing a lot bigger than he should be and when it came to delivering my baby he would be too big to deliver naturally. Two days before he was born the hospital predicted that he would weigh 9lb and they were spot on with his weight due to his measurements. I ended up electing for another caesarean section because I was worried he would get stuck if I tried to have a natural birth due to having gestational diabetes.

I ended up eating the same things day in and out. When not at work the best thing for me to eat for breakfast was protein which made my readings low. I ate bacon, egg, mushrooms and tomatoes. I was also surprised that eating various pies would give me a low reading. I had to avoid white food such as white bread, pasta and rice as these gave me a surge in readings. I got to a point where my readings were not low enough so the diabetic clinic put me on metformin. After taking this for a about a week I didn't feel very well. It gave me sweats in the night, a cracking headache, dry mouth and I felt generally unwell, but I didn't want to inject insulin because of the thought of using a needle. It was the best choice I then made going on to insulin because I felt better and it didn't hurt that much. Injecting twice a day through all this, I just tried to stay focused on why I was doing this and the benefits to myself and my baby. In this pregnancy I put on one stone and after the birth I was back to the weight I was before I got pregnant. I think this is due to having GDM and watching what I ate. **Zoe, GDM with second baby**

I hated the diabetes clinic. I felt like a number being processed. I rarely saw the same midwife as I had seen previously and got very sick of repeating my medical history over and over (no-one ever ever read my notes before speaking to me) and I was often told about what I was 'allowed' to do. It was a very stressful and unhappy experience. During late pregnancy when we began discussing the birth it got worse. My first child was born by emergency caesarean section and I was very much hoping for a VBAC. However, I was told that I would be induced and that I couldn't have a water birth. Obviously the additional risk of the previous section was also at play here. I was told about scary risks but not how likely they were or what the evidence was behind what they were telling me. I ended up in tears at this appointment, I didn't feel as though anyone was listening to me or cared about what I wanted. I also felt very vulnerable; I was being told all of this scary stuff without any understanding of the reasoning behind it, I simply didn't have enough information and felt unsupported. After this appointment I consulted with an independent midwife who was brilliant. She talked through my previous birth experience, looked at my blood sugar data, and found information for me including the latest midwifery journal articles relating to my situation. She was reassuring and supportive. She told me the actual risks in numerical terms and why. She saw no reason for my birth to be particularly risky. She came with me to my next consultant appointment and the consultant acted quite differently when she was there, and suddenly the water birth I wanted was not impossible. Following this appointment and after doing my own research into the risks, I decided how I wanted my birth to go and I wrote a letter to the consultant detailing what I would and wouldn't consent to. I felt as though I had to fight for the birth I wanted, so I did everything I could to make it happen. I went into labour naturally at 40 + 6 and had a successful VBAC in the pool. The labour midwives were great, very supportive, read my notes and birth plan before speaking to me, and helped me to have the birth I wanted. My daughter was not a particularly large baby.
Rebecca, GDM with second baby

I went in to be induced on my due date as I was advised that this was necessary with gestational diabetes. There were a series of unavoidable delays so I actually went into labour spontaneously which was great as I really didn't want to be induced. My baby was born naturally and was a hefty 10lb 9½oz. **Joanna, GDM with second baby**

I was induced at 39+1 and our 7lb 8oz baby boy arrived the following day with a natural vaginal birth. **Nicola, GDM with first baby**

I was booked in for an early induction (38 weeks) which thankfully went smoothly and my little boy was born weighing exactly 8lbs. I'd had some other complications during my pregnancy too so I was already high risk but, although I was unable to have a water birth as I was wired up with drips, my labour and birth were beautiful and I wouldn't change it. **Nicki, GDM with first baby**

No one ever discussed my birth or what would happen nearer to my due date. My trawl of the relatively few internet articles suggested that it wouldn't be possible for me to have the active water birth I had planned due to the Gestational Diabetes, and that most likely, I would be induced. But again, when I questioned this at my appointments I was met with a reluctance to discuss it. In the weeks that followed, I had regular hospital appointments and growth scans. Everything was always fine, and my blood sugar always remained normal. I had to take a lot of time off work for the appointments which only compounded the stress that I already felt. …At 37 weeks, I had my final growth scan which showed, if anything, that the baby was measuring slightly smaller than they might expect, though the sonographer assured me that growth scans for the weight of the baby can be inaccurate. I then went into an appointment with a junior consultant to 'book my induction'. Confused, I questioned why they would induce me when the baby wasn't measuring big, but was simply told it was standard procedure for women with Gestational Diabetes. "But I've never had a high reading since the original GTT" I retorted, "it doesn't make any sense and I would like to avoid unnecessary induction if possible." I was then sent to see a more senior consultant who spoke to me like I was a child and asked me did I know about the risk of still birth? I repeated my retort and the consultant finally said that they would review it again at 39-40 weeks. My baby cheated induction, and my son arrived naturally a week later at 38 weeks weighing 6lbs 1oz. It wasn't the active, water birth I wanted. His heartbeat was monitored throughout the labour, and I fought for this to happen standing up rather than lying down on a bed. Luckily, I had done an NCT course and had written a birth plan as part of that, so at least the midwives knew my wishes. Had this not been the case, at no point in my Gestational Diabetes care did anyone mention a birth plan. It seemed that with my diagnosis, I had also waived my right to choice. **Sophie, GDM with first baby**

Having had two particularly quick previous home births I felt it was in my best interests to go ahead with my planned home birth. I was supported in my choices by most of the birth professionals I came into contact with. I did have to remind some of them that it was my choice and their role was to advise and support me in my choice. I worked out a plan with my community midwife for managing the gestational diabetes both during the birth and after. I was happy to have my blood sugars monitored during labour and make decisions at the time. My son was born at home in water with an NHS midwife one afternoon. As expected my active labour was very short and the midwife only just made it in time. She barely had time to check my sugar levels when she arrived before baby was born! I only had one midwife present (same as my other two labours) because of the swiftness of my births. If I had planned to go to the hospital I probably would not have made it in time as from when I called the midwife to come to when he was born was only about an hour!

My first two children had been 2.8kgs and 3.86kgs and birthed easily using my hypnobirthing skills. My third (and last) was 4.3kgs. He was the slowest of all my second stages (although only a few minutes) and with an intact perineum. All in all I was mostly supported in my choice but did need to be quite firm at times and found it emotionally quite stressful to be going outside of the guidelines and be met with some resistance. Luckily I am quite confident and able to speak up for myself and achieved a wonderful calm and easy home birth. That is not to say that I didn't find it difficult to stick to my choices and there were moments when I doubted myself and felt very much alone in making decisions for myself and my baby. **Soshanna, GDM with third baby**

Chapter 5:
Postnatal Care - the first few days

Looking after yourself

For the first day or two, continue to monitor your blood glucose and eat as advised by your dietitian during pregnancy. Your family will probably be delighted to bring you nutritious snacks – tell them what you want them to bring beforehand. Your blood glucose will almost certainly return to normal pre-pregnancy levels within this time, and you should test that this is so before you go home if you give birth in hospital.

If you have been on any therapy to lower your plasma glucose levels, then you can stop this immediately after you have given birth. However do be aware of the symptoms of high plasma glucose and seek medical advice or ring your specialist team if you suspect that your glucose levels are high (these are listed in Chapter3).

Make sure you know how your GDM will be followed up (more on this in the next chapter) before you are discharged from midwifery care. Chapter 6 will discuss prevention of both GDM in future pregnancies (you are more likely to have GDM in future pregnancies once you have had it once) and later type 2 diabetes, but some information on both of these should be made available to you before you are discharged from midwifery care.

Feeding your baby and managing newborn hypoglycaemia

Breastfeeding reduces the chance of a child developing diabetes later in life, as well as having many other health benefits. Breastfeeding also has many benefits to you as it has an impact on a woman's metabolism and postnatal weight loss. I discuss its benefits in regard to diabetes prevention in Chapter 6, and there are many good sources of information available on its many extensive health benefits to mother and baby. If you are planning to feed your baby formula milk, then you might want to review your decision in light of your GDM and the possible effects on both you and your child in preventing future diabetes. As well as the benefits of breastfeeding, there are also the health disadvantages of formula-milk to consider: cow's milk protein may play a role in the development of type 1 diabetes in susceptible children (InFact, 2006).

Giving your baby formula milk not only means that your body does not receive the protection that lactation over a period of time provides (such as reduced diabetes rate, improved weight loss, reduced breast cancer rate) but it also means that your baby is exposed to a substance that does not boost his or her immune system, and that is more likely to lead to him or her becoming overweight or obese in later life, itself a risk for diabetes. Human milk has so many benefits over the modified cow's milk of formula, both for the mother who produces it and the baby who drinks it; diabetes prevention is just one of those benefits.

Whether you plan to feed your baby your own breastmilk or formula milk, early feeding can be particularly important when there has been GDM during pregnancy and should take place within the first 30 to 60 minutes. First, skin-to-skin contact after birth (baby lying on your chest and in direct contact with your skin or your partner's if you are unable to do this for any reason) will help your baby maintain his or her body temperature, and hence stabilise blood sugar, and stimulate the baby to feed. This immediate skin-to-skin contact should be uninterrupted, last as long as you and your baby want, and happen regardless of the way you intend to feed your baby.

Your baby will have been producing extra insulin whilst in your womb to help him or her use up the extra glucose going to him or her. This extra glucose is the reason why your baby may be a little bigger than others. However, once outside the comfort of your womb and your higher than normal blood glucose levels, it takes your baby a while to readjust his/her insulin output. Whilst it remains higher, it is likely that this extra insulin will cause your baby's glucose to be used up quicker and for him/her to develop low blood glucose or **hypoglycaemia**. The best way to prevent this is to feed baby as soon and as often as you can (at least every 2 to 3 hours as most babies do) in the first 24 to 48 hours.

You should be offered support to make sure you are able to get your baby to your breast as soon as you can. If you are planning to formula feed, have a bottle of formula milk to offer soon after the birth. Prompt feeding reduces the chance of **neonatal hypoglycaemia** (low blood sugars in your baby), and is a priority for you and your baby. The midwife should offer you help to feed your baby but if she is busy clearing up your birthing room or writing notes or doing things on a computer and you need or want assistance, then remind her (or ask your partner to remind her) that your baby needs to be fed and ask for help to feed him or her. If you are making a written birth plan, include this so that those looking after you also have it noted as a priority.

If you are going to breastfeed your baby, consider and discuss the possibility of expressing milk in late pregnancy and bringing this with you so that it can be fed to your baby by cup or spoon if he or she does not feed much early on for any reason. The Breastfeeding Network has an excellent section and a downloadable leaflet on Expressing and Storing Breastmilk in its Breastfeeding Information section (see resources section). Talk to your diabetes midwife or a breastfeeding counsellor or lactation consultant about expressing and the facilities for bringing in expressed breastmilk (often called EBM) with you to hospital. Do not be put off if you only express what appears to be a small amount of milk – say 1 to 5mls (up to a teaspoonful) of EBM – your baby's stomach is very small, about the size of a small walnut, and colostrum (the breastmilk in the first few days) is highly nutritious and well-absorbed so small amounts go a long way.

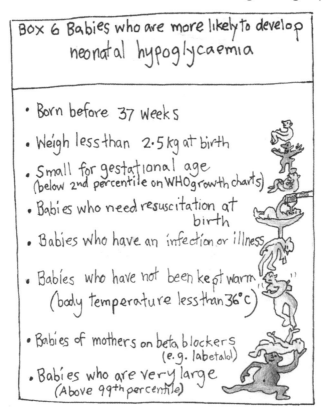

Box 6 Babies who are more likely to develop neonatal hypoglycaemia

- Born before 37 weeks
- Weigh less than 2.5 kg at birth
- Small for gestational age (below 2nd percentile on WHO growth charts)
- Babies who need resuscitation at birth
- Babies who have an infection or illness
- Babies who have not been kept warm (body temperature less than 36°c)
- Babies of mothers on beta blockers (e.g. labetalol)
- Babies who are very large (Above 99th percentile)

Whilst most babies of mothers with GDM do not develop hypoglycaemia, some do and it is difficult to identify which babies will do so (those who are <u>most likely</u> to become hypoglycaemic are listed in Box 6 above). It is therefore usual practice to monitor baby's blood glucose levels 2 to 4 hours after birth and to repeat this at intervals <u>before or at the start of feeds</u>, over at least 24 hours, until these are stable within the normal range (e.g. 2.6mmol/L or above for 3 consecutive readings). This means that you will be asked to allow your baby's heel to be pricked with a small lancet to draw enough blood to

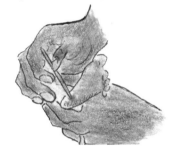

test (in much the same way you have been testing via your finger ends). It is known that babies are less disturbed by this if they are being fed or cuddled in their mother's arms (in fact babies who are being fed whilst it is done may appear not even to notice).

You have the right to decline consent for your baby to be tested in this way, and to ask for an alternative approach to assessing your baby's well-being. AIMS is aware that parents who do decline this or other tests can come under pressure from health professionals. However, discussing signs and symptoms (see illustrations below), and helping you to check on and feed your baby is an alternative. The AIMS helpline is also available for support and to talk things over.

If you do not want your baby's blood to be tested or are at home without facilities to do a test regularly, then the physical signs of newborn hypoglycaemia are shown in the illustration below. If you suspect your baby is hypoglycaemic, *whether or not your baby's blood has been tested*, seek the immediate assistance of a health professional

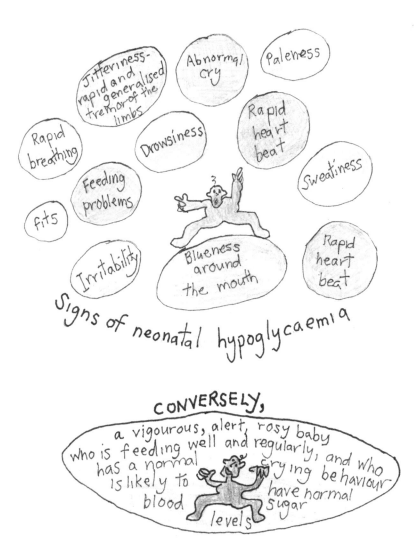

Signs of neonatal hypoglycaemia

Jitteriness - rapid and generalised tremor of the limbs

Abnormal cry

Paleness

Rapid breathing

Drowsiness

Rapid heart beat

Sweatiness

Feeding problems

Fits

Irritability

Blueness around the mouth

Rapid heart beat

CONVERSELY,

a vigourous, alert, rosy baby who is feeding well and regularly, and who has a normal crying behaviour is likely to have normal blood sugar levels

If baby's blood glucose is low (less than 2mmol/L), you will be asked to feed him or her. If you are breastfeeding and your baby is not yet feeding well from the breast, you can give him or her milk that you expressed before birth, if you have any, or you can hand express a little milk or use donor milk. If none of these options are available, then you may want to consider giving a little formula milk until you are in a position to give your own breastmilk. See the Resources section after Chapter 6 for links to more information on expressing breastmilk.

Hypoglycaemia in a baby can sometimes be a difficult situation to manage. Your baby needs to raise his/her blood glucose by feeding, but babies with low glucose can be sleepy and harder to latch onto the breast, and can sometimes not suckle well to start with. In this instance, expressing some of your milk may be very helpful. Often, just giving some expressed breastmilk can give them enough energy to start to breastfeed directly so it is worth trying just a few mls of expressed milk and then trying to feed at the breast again. If this doesn't work, consider giving a full feed of expressed milk and then try again at the breast. It's really worthwhile finding and contacting a certified breastfeeding counsellor in advance and asking them for support if you are working through these initial challenges.

As time will be pressing if your baby's blood sugars are low, having standby expressed breastmilk ready will really help. But this isn't always possible and some mothers do decide to give formula in this situation, if only on one occasion. If you are giving either expressed breastmilk or formula but are planning to breastfeed, ask to be shown how to feed by cup, syringe or spoon instead of using a bottle. Feeding by bottle can interfere with some babies' latching onto the breast in the early days, as the way that they latch to a bottle (no matter what the bottle company says about its product being close to a natural breast shape) is different to the way they latch to the breast. Most babies feed very well indeed from a cup and midwives often use small medicine cups to feed babies; they can show you how to do this. There are lots of YouTube clips showing babies cup feeding.

If you are breastfeeding but have decided to give formula, remember your baby does not need as much formula as a bottle-fed baby. Giving too much will make the baby full and uninterested in the breast, and it is important that the baby suckles regularly to stimulate your milk supply. A rough guide for how much formula milk to give to a breastfed baby in this situation is 30mls per kg per 24 hours at about 3-hourly intervals (8 feeds per 24 hours) so a baby weighing 3kg would need 90mls/8=11.25mls per feed. So beware of being given a whole 100ml bottle of milk. Ask for the correct amount to be poured into a cup instead. (Babies need more formula than they would of EBM because the body is unable to digest the formula as efficiently as it does breastmilk.)

Once your baby's blood glucose is stable, continue to make sure your baby is fed frequently, at least 10 to 12 times over the following 24 hours, and spend as much time in skin-to-skin contact as you can as this will continue to help your baby maintain both body temperature and blood glucose levels, as well as all the other benefits (Moore *et al.*, 2012).

Babies whose mothers have had GDM are also slightly more likely to have **neonatal jaundice**. If there are signs of jaundice, such as an increasing yellow tinge to the skin and eye whites, then this may also involve blood tests for **bilirubin** levels and treatment under blue light if the levels are high. If you are already home (jaundice tends to develop from day 3 or 4), then your community midwife will monitor and advise you but, if you think your baby is developing jaundice, feed him or her frequently and place in daylight (though not in direct sunshine). Feeding your baby helps to flush out the bilirubin via the digestive tract into his or her stools. Inform your community midwife and ask for a visit if one isn't already scheduled.

If your baby needs special care on a neonatal unit

If your baby's blood glucose remains low or unstable (below 2.0mmol/L on two consecutive readings despite support with feeding), he or she may be transferred to a special neonatal unit for closer monitoring, and possibly tube-feeding or, more rarely, intravenous dextrose infusion (NICE, 2015). Tube-feeding is where a thin tube is passed into baby's stomach via his/her nose and milk (EBM or formula) can be fed through it. Intravenous infusions are when fluid is delivered directly into the blood stream through very small tubing. This tubing is attached to a cannula (also a small plastic tube which sits in the baby's vein and is introduced by a tiny needle). These are both too complicated to do or manage on a postnatal ward and are better done in the neonatal unit, which has much tighter infection control and staff well-trained in and adept at using these techniques. Your agreement and consent should be sought before anything is done to your baby (except in an emergency, when it will be presumed, unless you say otherwise), so do make sure you get all the information you want during these discussions.

You and the baby's father will be able to visit at all times but this can be difficult if, for example, you had a caesarean birth and are still relatively immobile. You should be able to be provided with a wheelchair so that someone can take you to see your baby as soon as possible. Often neonatal units are on a different floor to the postnatal ward and this means you may lose out on midwifery postnatal care and support or even meals if you are absent from your ward for long periods. Talk to the midwife looking after you and liaise with her about when you will be available for a talk and check-up, and what you want to do about meals.

Neonatal ward staff are often, though not always, very good at explaining your baby's care but they will largely see you as a visitor (albeit a very important one!) and not as a 'patient'. This can be difficult in the first couple of days after having a baby, when YOU need a lot of looking after whatever sort of birth you had. Remember to drink plenty of fluids and rest as much as you can – sometimes you may need to leave your partner or mother with your baby while you go and lie down for an hour or so.

A baby's temporary stay on a neonatal unit in a situation like this can be very tiring, upsetting and disorientating as it breaks up your getting-to-know-each-other time, however well managed and short-term. This often coincides with the period in which you may experience the so-called 'baby blues' (a few days in which you can feel emotionally fragile or weepy as your hormones readjust, usually around the 2nd to 5th postnatal day). So be patient with yourself and seek support – this is a temporary situation, it is not your fault and your baby needs your love and touch; talking to your baby and stroking him or her, or having your baby in skin-to-skin care (often known on neonatal units as 'kangaroo care') will help and comfort you both and strengthen your growing relationship, as well as help breastfeeding and stabilisation of baby's temperature control and heart-rate.

Womens' Experiences

Our baby girl was born peacefully at home (VBAC) in a birth pool, we weren't apart from each other at all, so we had the most wonderful skin-to-skin bonding time together (a complete contrast to my first daughter's birth). Then one of the midwives (this particular midwife had just arrived after the birth) said that I needed to make sure our daughter fed soon in order to do the blood sugar test; then I felt the pressure for our baby to attach and feed. I had been a breastfeeding peer supporter, and knew from my training that a baby doesn't 'need' to feed straight away as they are sustained by what they received whilst in the womb, and in some cases babies may take some hours to feed, so I hadn't been worried and wanted to just let our baby girl lay with me all snuggled up warm and let her find her own way, in her own time. I felt the pressure to see her attach and feed, but why did I let this pressure get to me, I knew she was ok, I knew my blood sugars were fine and so wouldn't have spiked hers. It came to the 2 hours and she still hadn't fed, so the midwife said she'd take her blood sugar level anyway and it was absolutely fine. Phew! No need to go into hospital. We were told the signs to look out for should there be a change in her blood sugar levels, but all was fine. **Stacey, GDM with second baby**

My son had a plump tummy due to the diabetes but his sugar levels were absolutely fine, we were both monitored throughout the first night. **Nicola, GDM with second baby**

My baby's blood sugar was checked after the birth, and then no one mentioned diabetes again. As quickly as it started, my episode with Gestational Diabetes had ended. How had it made me feel? Upset, panicked, frustrated, restricted, exhausted from fighting for everything I wanted for so many weeks... I could go on. In short, the stress from it ruined the last 11 weeks of my pregnancy - the constant testing, scans and appointments. I often wonder whether it contributed to the early arrival of my son. I'll never know. Despite a fairly straightforward birth, I ended up staying in hospital for a week due to my baby struggling to feed and being deemed 'too small'. The stress only ended when he was six weeks old and finally managed to latch and I had a final OGTT - the readings were fine, no surprise. **Sophie, GDM with first baby**

My levels returned to normal literally immediately. My son's levels were slightly low on the first two readings but soon came up and did not cause us to stay in hospital much longer than we would've anyway. **Nicola, GDM with first baby**

My baby had blood sugars that were a little bit low but not so as to cause the medics any concerns, and after a bit of breastfeeding they soon stabilised; I really didn't want to give top-ups. The only thing that I was annoyed about afterwards was when I found out that I should have been spoken to about expressing colostrum towards the end of the pregnancy, which might have helped stabilise his blood sugars earlier. **Nicki, GDM with first baby**

Once my baby was born he was monitored for the first 24 hours and his blood sugar levels checked before each feed. Luckily he has not been affected. **Zoe, GDM with second baby**

I found it frustrating to have to speak to the consultant on the phone after just having had a baby at home and reiterate that I was happy to monitor my baby myself at home and did not feel the need to go in, which is what had already been discussed and planned at my home birth meeting at 36 weeks. The midwife was fantastic. She returned to check baby's sugar levels later that evening (baby was born in the afternoon) and again the following morning. She left me with clear instructions of what to look for, what to do and to call 999 if I was concerned at all. I planned to breastfeed (having successfully breastfed my other two children) and was happy to monitor him through the night offering him the breast more frequently and not letting him go for longer than 4 hours without a feed. I had harvested colostrum on the last few weeks of my pregnancy, should my new baby need any help stabilising his sugar levels, as I did not want him to have formula unnecessarily. I had over 25 x 5ml colostrum feeds in the freezer ready for if I needed it. **Soshanna, GDM with third baby**

Chapter 6:
Preventing Diabetes after GDM

What should I do after I have had GDM?
What are the longer-term implications of GDM?

Let's first consider what happens shortly after your GDM-affected pregnancy and the follow-up care you should expect.

Testing plasma glucose levels after having GDM and what the results mean

Nearly everyone whose insulin-resistance in pregnancy has led to high plasma glucose and a diagnosis of GDM goes back to having normal plasma glucose after their baby is born. In other words, once pregnancy ends, women who had GDM are no longer 'diabetic'. All daily testing and treatment of the mother stops at or shortly after birth (the baby may continue to require extra blood tests and observation for 48 hours), and life goes back to normal as far as it can with a new baby!

All women who have had GDM should be offered a follow-up blood test about 6 to 13 weeks postnatally. This is usually a fasting plasma glucose test to confirm that glucose metabolism has returned to normal and type 2 diabetes has not developed (NICE, 2015).

Each year, you should be invited by your GP practice for a further blood test to check that all is well and you have not developed type 2 diabetes. These annual tests usually consist of a single blood test called HbA1c (H-B-A-one-C). The HbA1c test shows what your average plasma glucose has been over the previous 2 to 3 months and, if it is high, will indicate whether further tests are required. It is occasionally used in the initial postnatal check at 6 to 13 weeks instead of a fasting plasma glucose test.

However not every woman who needs this follow-up is offered it (usually through simple administrative error) so if you think you haven't been offered a follow-up appointment, do chase it up if you want the test. Also, make sure your GP is aware if you have had GDM and that you are invited for a yearly review appointment (this will probably be with a practice nurse) if you want annual testing.

One third of women who have had GDM do not attend any follow-up appointments, either because they haven't received an appointment or because they have decided not to attend. Of course, you may choose not to go to any follow-up appointments but do stay alert for the signs of diabetes listed in Chapter 3. Undiagnosed and therefore untreated diabetes can have a serious impact on health and some mothers go on to develop type 2 diabetes without realising it, until they are feeling quite ill with the symptoms of high plasma glucose.

If your fasting plasma glucose at 6 to 13 weeks after your baby's birth is 6.0 to 6.9mmol/L (or 39 to 47mmol/mol if you have had an HbA1c test), then you are at a greater risk of developing type 2 diabetes in the future than if it is lower (NICE, 2015). If your fasting plasma glucose is over 7.0mmol/L (or above 48mmol/mol if you have had an HbA1c test), it is likely that you already have diabetes (nearly always type 2 diabetes) and will be offered tests to confirm this.

There is much current discussion and interest in work showing that type 2 diabetes can be reversed through diet. See, for example, Dr David Cavan's books *Reverse Your Diabetes* and *Reverse Your Diabetes Diet*, both of which are widely available. There are many positive reports and research results emerging about using dietary changes to reverse type 2 diabetes – some of this work can be viewed at *www.ncl.ac.uk/magres/research/diabetes/reversal.htm*.

Preventing type 2 diabetes after having GDM: breastfeeding, lifestyle change, drug therapy

NICE recommends that all women with GDM are offered lifestyle advice (weight control, diet, exercise) after their GDM pregnancy. The aim of this advice is to prevent a recurrence in a subsequent pregnancy and to prevent the later development of type 2 diabetes.

One of the reasons there is so much medical and scientific interest in GDM is because it is closely associated with the development of type 2 diabetes later in life, both in the women affected and the children born from the affected pregnancy as they grow up. About 12% of women develop type 2 diabetes in the 2 years following their GDM pregnancy (Gunderson et al., 2015), and 30% to 50% of women develop type 2 diabetes within 5 to 10 years of the affected pregnancy, with some studies reporting rates of over 60% (Lee et al., 2007; Zeigler et al., 2012; Ignell et al., 2016, Rayanagoudar et al., 2016).

A systematic review of research has looked at who is most likely to go on to develop type 2 diabetes after a GDM pregnancy (Rayanagoudar et al., 2016). The following GDM-pregnancy factors were found to be associated with future type 2 diabetes: higher plasma glucose levels, need for insulin, earlier onset of GDM, and BMI above 25 being most predictive; preterm birth (before 37 weeks gestation), high blood pressure in the GDM pregnancy, a family history of diabetes, and non-white ethnicity having moderate effect; and being over 30 years of age and multiparity having a smaller effect. Women whose body fat is greater in the upper body (apple-shape) are thought to be more likely to develop diabetes than women whose fat is lower down (pear-shape). (Poston, 2016)

Type 2 diabetes is associated with cardiac, renal, circulation and eyesight problems, all of which develop over a number of years, depending on how well (or not) plasma glucose is controlled. These problems tend to worsen the longer someone has diabetes. So, whilst developing type 2 diabetes in your seventies or eighties may not lead to chronic illness or a serious shortening of life (there just isn't enough time for it to do this), early development of type 2 diabetes, which is seen more commonly nowadays, does mean that the chronic illnesses associated with it (renal failure, poor circulation to the legs and feet, eyesight problems, heart disease) can have an adverse effect on the quality and length of life of people who develop it. This is why there is so much research into preventing both GDM and type 2 diabetes, and also, importantly, preventing type 2 diabetes in women who have had GDM.

Breastfeeding

Women with GDM were followed up for two years in a recent study and those who breastfed most (that is breastfed for longer than 2 months and gave only or mostly breastmilk to their babies) were approximately 50% less likely to have developed type 2 diabetes by the time their babies were two years old (Gunderson *et al.*, 2015). This gives added weight to earlier findings that:

Breastfeeding by women who had GDM was associated with a >40% long-term reduction of the risk of developing postpartum diabetes. Risk reduction was most pronounced when lactation was continued for at least 3 months, and the beneficial effects of lactation on diabetes risk were sustained over time. (Zeigler *et al.*, 2012)

The reason for this appears to be that breastfeeding leads to improvements in insulin sensitivity, glucose uptake by body cells, and some other key metabolic pathways associated with type 2 diabetes (Gunderson *et al.*, 2015; Much *et al.*, 2016).

For help and support with longer-term breastfeeding, look for a Baby Café or La Leche League group or breastfeeding specialist or lactation consultant in your area. If your family and friends are unsure about or uncomfortable with the idea of you breastfeeding your baby beyond the first few weeks, it will be very important for you to have the support of other mothers and your midwife and health visitor, and to explain to your friends and family why this is important for your health as well as your baby's. Some breastfeeding support groups are listed in the resource section near the end of the book.

Lifestyle change

The other best way that is known to diminish the chance of developing type 2 diabetes is weight loss and exercise (DUK, 2011; NIHR, 2016). Weight loss means a reduction in body fat because this reduces insulin-resistance and, as a consequence, plasma glucose levels. Even relatively small amounts of weight loss, say 5% of your weight which is 5kg if you weigh 100kg (or 11 lbs if you weigh 220lbs), can make a difference. The 'risk-factor' for type 2 diabetes that is most modifiable or able to be changed is body weight and nearly all advice you receive will reiterate this. Exercise is also important, first because it helps with weight loss but also because it is beneficial whether or not you lose weight. Exercise builds muscle mass, which reduces overall insulin-resistance by using insulin more effectively than fat.

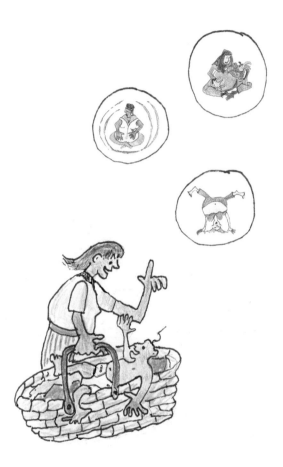

There are currently research studies looking at specific lifestyle changes that help women who have had GDM avoid developing type 2 diabetes. Those that have been done have used a variety of interventions in various combinations. Some have reported a reduction in the development of type 2 diabetes by between a third and two-thirds through lifestyle changes such as:

* reducing fat intake
* increasing fibre-intake
* reducing calorie-intake
* taking moderate exercise for 2.5 to 4 hours a week
* reducing body-weight by 5 to 7%
* working with a lifestyle counsellor monthly to change lifestyle

Two **systematic reviews** found that there is research evidence for the effectiveness of lifestyle change (either dietary changes, increased physical activity or both) in preventing type 2 diabetes after GDM, though some studies had problems recruiting sufficient women (Morton et al., 2014; Gilinsky et al., 2015). A recent study from the USA's huge Diabetes Prevention Program found both lifestyle change and metformin (see below) were effective in reducing progression to diabetes during a 10-year follow-up period (Aroda et al., 2015). Similar prevention programmes are becoming widely available in the UK, and your GP or practice nurse may know of one near you.

There is also good evidence, in relation to type 2 diabetes prevention across the wider population, that lifestyle change aimed at reducing BMI and increasing exercise is a good idea if you have had GDM (Unwin and Unwin, 2014). Whilst it will not guarantee that you avoid diabetes, it will certainly make it less likely that you do develop it or it will delay its development (Lancet 2006). Ignell and colleagues followed up 362 women after a GDM pregnancy in Sweden (Ignell et al., 2016). They found that BMI was closely associated with an increased likelihood of developing diabetes after a GDM pregnancy. But BMI can be reduced and this may be the most important way of preventing type 2 diabetes.

Your GP or practice nurse will be able to help and advise you about making lifestyle changes and support you in this, or be able to signpost you to activities or practitioners in your area. Other mothers on social media may be able to advise you about local groups and facilities that are best geared towards those with a young baby in tow. Making lifestyle changes during the topsy-turvy time with a new baby and small children can be difficult – the practicalities of getting anywhere with a baby/toddler, tiredness and having less income all make getting exercise, shopping and food preparation more challenging. Joining with other mothers can give the support and encouragement that makes it all do-able or even enjoyable. If the first thing you try doesn't suit you, do keep trying to find something that suits you better.

Drugs

Some researchers, as already mentioned, have studied whether drugs can play a role in preventing the development of type 2 diabetes. Metformin (the drug most commonly used to treat type 2 diabetes) has been found to reduce the rate of type 2 diabetes after GDM. However, there is no simple route to preventing diabetes. For example, metformin causes gastro-intestinal side-effects in some people, and the researchers estimated that many women need to take the drug for a few years to avoid developing type 2 diabetes:

In a number-needed-to-treat analysis, the study found seven women with GDM would need to receive metformin to prevent one case of type 2 diabetes within 10 years. (Aroda, 2015)

In terms of health benefit, this sort of treatment to benefit ratio (7:1) is judged worthwhile by health service planners, but you may decide that the 1 in 7 chance of benefit to you personally is not so acceptable.

Breastfeeding, lifestyle change and, for some, taking metformin all have a role to play in reducing diabetes after GDM or delaying its onset. You can reduce the chance of becoming diabetic by taking action, and then look forward to healthy grandmotherhood as well as motherhood!

Women's Experiences

My diabetes disappeared straight away and I have annual checks to make sure I am avoiding type 2 diabetes. I arrange these myself at the GP's. Although I was told I would need these checks, it is up to me to remember to arrange them. I understand that my son is at an increased risk of type 2 diabetes, which we will need to be aware of and make him aware as he gets older. He is 2 now. I have been warned that I am very likely to get gestational diabetes again so I plan to give up sugar completely before attempting to conceive again to give myself and any future babies the best chance. **Joanna, GDM with second baby**

Nothing has been mentioned about my diabetes since the birth. I don't know if I still have it. So I have to wait anxiously till my 6 week check up with my doctor to see if I have managed to get rid of this. The diabetic clinic have told me I have a 50% chance of getting diabetes in later life anyway and suggested I need to reduce my BMI asap. This is not an easy challenge after having a caesarean section and with a newborn baby on 3 hourly feeds. I have started to crave sugar again since he was born to keep my energy levels up for the 3 night feeds. They completely sap your energy! I am just glad to no longer have to inject insulin and I hope at my check-up that diabetes is all clear. I live in hope. It has been an eye opening experience. I am still shocked at the amount of sugars in food and drink products, but it has made me more aware! **Zoe, GDM with second baby**

E-resources and Social Media

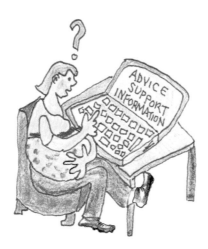

1. The Association for Improvements in Maternity Services (AIMS): *www.aims.org.uk*

Information and support on all matters relating to pregnancy and birth, the maternity services, and choices and rights relating to these.

Helpline email : *helpline@aims.org.uk*.   This email will go to a group of AIMS volunteers and someone will respond as soon as possible.

Telephone: 0300 365 0663: This phone number will connect you to an AIMS volunteer when possible, otherwise leave a message and someone will get back to you.

(Calls to 03 numbers cost no more than a national rate call and will be covered by phone contract inclusive minutes in the same way as 01 and 02 calls.)

2. Women with Gestational Diabetes website

This website has lots of information presented in a series of short video clips mainly of women talking about their experiences of having GDM, along with some health professional input and some useful diagrammatic illustrations. It outlines the standard care offered and is occasionally prescriptive e.g. "you will have to attend.....". But it is also largely sensible and positive. There are interactive elements such as quizzes, and some practical guides with more in depth information e.g. on insulin. ***www.womenwithgestationaldiabetes.com***

3. Gestational Diabetes UK Mums: website and social media forums

An informative website run by a GDM mother with loads of useful information including meal plans, drug guides, borderline diagnoses, and excellent sections on induction, and choosing water birth or homebirth. There is so much on this website and it also has links to policy and research documents. Some of the pages (e.g. meal guides) are accessible only through membership which stands currently (2017) at £5 (bronze) or £7 (silver) a month. But most of the website is accessible for free. ***www.gestationaldiabetes.co.uk***

Gestational Diabetes UK Mums can also be followed via:

Twitter: @GDUKMums
Instagram: @gestational_diabetes_uk
Facebook: Gestational Diabetes UK Mums

4. Pregnant with Diabetes App

This free app from a team in Copenhagen and designed by a woman with diabetes is available in English or Danish. It covers all basic information clearly. It is available widely, including on iTunes.

(There are a number of other GDM apps available at a cost but many of these are from the USA and the information may be hard to apply to other countries.)

5.   Management of Hyperglycaemia in Pregnancy

This well-produced and easy to follow web-based course outlines nutrition and food choices in a GDM pregnancy. It is informative, interactive and interesting but does come from the USA so some allowances for language and practices have to be made.

http://learntelehealth.org/modules/
ManagementGestationalDiabetesOutput/story.html

6.   Some websites asking or attempting to answer key questions about GDM (they are from USA so do allow for the many differences in health care approaches)

This one is written by a woman who had GDM and who did end up needing insulin:

http://birthwithoutfearblog.com/2013/06/24/the-truth-about-
gestational-diabetes-and-why-its-not-your-fault

This is a site trying to answer questions about induction of labour:

http://evidencebasedbirth.com/does-gestational-diabetes-
always-mean-a-big-baby-and-induction/

This is the consensus statement from the National Institutes of Health on Diagnosing GDM:

*https://consensus.nih.gov/2013/docs/Gestational_Diabetes_*
Mellitus508.pdf

7.   Polycystic Ovary Syndrome

Verity is a self-help group for women with polycystic ovary syndrome (PCOS). *www.verity-pcos.org.uk*

8.   Glycaemic Index Tables

I have chosen some fairly comprehensive but simple tables below. The Diabetes UK website (no. 10 below), and the University of Sydney's GI unit (**www.glycemicindex.com**) have much more comprehensive but complex information if you want to explore further. **www.the-gi-diet.org/glycemicindexchart**

www.weightlossresources.co.uk/diet/gi_diet/glycaemic_index_ tables.htm

9.   Breastfeeding and expressing breastmilk

The Breastfeeding Network and The Association of Breastfeeding Mothers both have excellent downloadable leaflets on expressing and storing breastmilk – look in the Breastfeeding Information sections. The ABM one is also available in Spanish.

www.breastfeedingnetwork.org.uk (also telephone and online support).

http://abm.me.uk

www.thebaby.org/your-nearest-baby-cafe.html – find your nearest Baby Café.

www.laleche.org.uk/find-lll-support-group - find your nearest LLL group.

Information on recognising and responding to feeding cues and lots more useful information about feeding in the first days: **http://kellymom.com/bf/normal/hunger-cues**

10. Diabetes UK (DUK): *www.diabetes.org.uk*

The main UK charity for people living with diabetes. DUK has an extensive website and produces many resources. It produces a booklet on Gestational Diabetes that contains useful information on reading food labels, injecting insulin, testing your blood glucose and lifestyle advice. DUK also has a weekday **helpline** (0345 123 2399) and email help facility (**careline@diabetes.org.uk**).

11. Lifestyle apps

There are a wide number of apps available to support lifestyle change:

The **NHS** has a range of free apps for healthy eating, exercise, alcohol awareness and smoking cessation on its <u>One You</u> website: ***www.nhs.uk/oneyou/apps***

Bounts has an app that offers you incentives to get active in the form of 'bounts', reward points that be turned into cash or vouchers. Joining is free: ***www.bounts.it***

My Fitness Pal has a range of tools and apps (free) to help people lose weight, such as food diaries, a food database, discussion forum, apps and activity logs: ***www.myfitnesspal.com***

Carbs and Cals is a key producer of tools (books and apps) for counting carbohydrates and calories using thousands of photos of food portions, with the nutritional info shown for each photo. Used by many health care professionals. Not free, apart from access to 50 downloadable, useful and interesting pdfs, but well worth a look: ***www.carbsandcals.com***

12. Film on gestational diabetes and lifestyle change to prevent type 2 diabetes

This lovely film from St. Lucia features a woman with GDM and her subsequent postnatal decisions around trying to prevent type 2 diabetes, and another who had undiagnosed type 2 diabetes. 22 minutes long, informative, moving and charming, the content is equally applicable to the UK. ***www.medicalaidfilms.org/film/diabetes***

Glossary

Bilirubin: a yellow pigment produced during normal breakdown of red blood cells which is processed by the liver, from where it is got rid of through the intestinal tract. A newborn baby's liver may not be mature enough to remove bilirubin efficiently so it accumulates in the body and causes jaundice (see neonatal jaundice below). Babies break down many of their red blood cells after birth as they do not need so many once born, hence why jaundice is common in newborn babies.

Birth injury: an injury caused by the birth process, usually due to birth attendants performing extra interventions to help the mother get the baby born e.g. in shoulder dystocia (see below). Injuries to babies can include cuts, bruising, and fractures, particularly of the collar bone or upper arm.

BMI/Body Mass Index: a measure of body fat depending on height and weight and calculated by multiplying weight in kilograms by height in metres squared (kg/m^2). This is a better indication of fatness than simply weight alone. BMI above $25kg/m^2$ denotes being overweight, and above $30kg/m^2$ indicates obesity or body fat likely to affect health.

Carbohydrates: Carbohydrates are sugars and starches, which, once changed by the body to glucose, provide energy. There are two types of carbohydrates, simple (or monosaccharides), and complex (or polysaccharides). Simple carbohydrates are found in fruits, dairy products, and processed, refined foods such as white sugar, pastas, and white bread. They are easily digested by the body, turned into glucose and quickly used up for energy, causing peaks and troughs in blood glucose levels. Complex carbohydrates take longer for the body to digest and are found in vegetables, wholegrain breads and pasta, brown rice, and pulses. Eating complex carbohydrates provides longer lasting energy and more stable blood sugar levels due to the slower way the body processes and uses the carbohydrates.

GDM/Gestational diabetes mellitus: Gestational diabetes also known as gestational diabetes mellitus or GDM, is a condition in which women without previously diagnosed diabetes exhibit high blood glucose levels during pregnancy.

Glucose: a simple sugar that provides the body with its primary source of energy. It is made by digesting and converting carbohydrates into a chemical form that the body can use as fuel.

Gestational Weight Gain: the amount of weight a woman gains during pregnancy, often abbreviated to GWG.

Glycaemic index (high/low): is a ranking of carbohydrate-containing foods based on the overall effect on blood glucose levels. Slowly absorbed foods have a low GI rating, while foods that are more quickly absorbed have a higher rating.

HbA1c: refers to *glycated haemoglobin* which identifies average plasma glucose concentration.

Hyperglycaemia: a condition in which an excessive amount of glucose circulates in the blood plasma (sometimes referred to as 'high blood sugar').

Hyperinsulinaemia: a condition in which there are excess levels of insulin circulating in the blood relative to the level of glucose. Hyperinsulinemia can be seen in a variety of conditions including type 2 diabetes mellitus and in newborn babies.

Hypertensive disorders of pregnancy: a group of disorders involving high blood pressure during pregnancy that includes chronic (pre-existing) hypertension, pre-eclampsia (see below) and eclampsia, pre-eclampsia superimposed on chronic hypertension, and gestational hypertension (transient hypertension in pregnancy or chronic hypertension identified in the latter half of pregnancy).

Hypoglycaemia: when blood glucose decreases to below normal levels. This can result in a variety of symptoms including clumsiness, trouble talking, confusion, loss of consciousness, seizures, or death (also known as 'low blood sugar').

IADPSG/International Diabetes in Pregnancy Study Group: a group of specialist doctors and scientists that aims to promote research and knowledge around diabetes and pregnancy.

Insulin: a hormone produced by beta cells of the pancreas that has important effects on the metabolism of carbohydrates, fats and protein by promoting the absorption of glucose from the blood into fat, liver and skeletal muscle cells. In these tissues the absorbed glucose is converted into glycogen or fats.

Insulin resistance: a condition in which body cells fail to respond to the normal actions of insulin. The body produces insulin when glucose starts to be released into the bloodstream from the digestion of carbohydrates. This insulin response triggers glucose being taken into body cells, to be used for energy. The level of glucose in the blood decreases as a result, staying within the normal range even when a large amount of carbohydrate is consumed. Under conditions of insulin resistance, the cells in the body are unable to use insulin as effectively, leading to high blood sugar. Beta cells in the pancreas subsequently increase their production of insulin, further contributing to a high blood insulin level. Insulin resistance naturally increases during pregnancy, probably to ensure the fetal brain receives enough glucose, and also, more generally, with increased body weight and fat accumulation.

Macrosomia: excessive birth weight, usually taken as being over the 90th percentile which is 4kg (8lb 13oz) for girls and 4.12kg (9lbs 1 oz) for boys at 40 weeks gestation amongst white European populations. Macrosomia, by definition, affects around 10% of pregnancies but is more common in pregnancies affected by GDM and diabetes.

Metformin: the most widely used medication for the treatment of type 2 diabetes, particularly in overweight people since it is not associated with weight gain, and has been in use for 60 years. Metformin is a biguanide and works by decreasing glucose production by the liver and increasing glucose use by body tissues. It is also used in the treatment of polycystic ovary syndrome. Common side effects include diarrhoea, nausea and abdominal discomfort and it is contraindicated in liver or renal disease.

Mmol/L: means millimoles per litre of blood and is how blood glucose levels are usually measured in the UK.

Neonatal hypoglycaemia: decreased blood glucose in a baby during the first 28 days. Untreated neonatal hypoglycaemia may result in brain injury that could lead to developmental problems later in life. It is the most common metabolic problem in newborns. Treatment is by immediate feeding by the most appropriate method (by mouth, naso-gastric tube or IV fluids) according to the baby's condition.

Neonatal jaundice: a yellowing of a baby's skin and eyes. Newborn jaundice is very common and can occur when babies have a high level of bilirubin (see above).

NICE/National Institute for Health and Care Excellence: a public body of the Department of Health serving both NHS England and NHS Wales set up in 1999. It publishes guidelines for health and social care based on research findings, with the aim of standardising and improving care, including guidelines for diabetes in pregnancy (www.nice. org.uk).

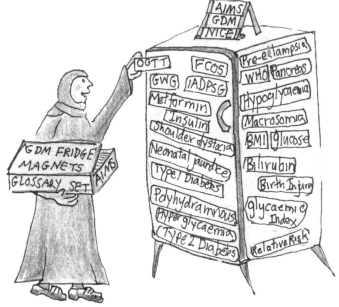

OGTT/oral glucose tolerance test: a test in which glucose is given and blood samples taken afterward to determine how quickly it is cleared from the blood. It is usually used to test for diabetes, insulin resistance, impaired pancreatic function, or rarer disorders of carbohydrate metabolism. A standard dose of glucose is taken by mouth and blood levels are checked one and/or two hours later. Variations of the OGTT exist with different doses of glucose and different intervals of sampling.

Pancreas: an organ of the digestive and endocrine systems located in the abdomen. It produces several important hormones, including insulin, which circulate in the blood. The pancreas is also a digestive organ, secreting pancreatic juice that assists digestion and absorption of nutrients.

Polycystic ovary syndrome /PCOS: a set of symptoms resulting from elevated male hormone in women. Signs and symptoms include irregular or no menstrual periods, heavy periods, excess body and facial hair, acne, pelvic pain, difficulty getting pregnant, and patches of thick, darker, velvety skin. Associated conditions include type 2 diabetes, obesity, obstructive sleep apnoea, heart disease, mood swings, and endometrial cancer.

Polyhydramnios: an excess of amniotic fluid in the pregnant womb. It is seen in about 1% of pregnancies. It is associated with an increased risk of various problems, including preterm birth, placental abruption, and fetal abnormalities, but can be benign. It is suspected when uterine size is large for gestational age. Ultrasound examination can confirm the diagnosis by estimating fluid amount.

Pre-eclampsia: a disorder of pregnancy and the early postnatal period characterised by high blood pressure and protein in the urine. It is also referred to as PET or, perhaps by your grandmother, as 'toxaemia'. It usually occurs in the third trimester of pregnancy and generally worsens over time. In severe PET there may be red blood cell breakdown, a low blood platelet count, impaired liver function, kidney dysfunction, swelling, shortness of breath due to fluid in the lungs, or visual disturbances. If left untreated, it may result in seizures at which point it is known as eclampsia.

Risk: the probability of suffering harm; the likelihood of experiencing a poor outcome; the difference in the risk for individuals with a factor as opposed to those in whom the factor is absent; the ratio of the incidence rate among individuals with a given risk factor to the incidence rate among those without it (relative risk). This is an important concept in maternity (as in all health) care. Risk is often conveyed as a certain, very probable or inevitable outcome of a 'risk factor' whereas it is usually only a possible, or somewhat more probable, outcome.

Shoulder dystocia: an obstruction of labour after the birth of the baby's head when the baby's anterior shoulder cannot pass below, or requires significant manipulation to pass below, the pubic symphysis. It is diagnosed when the baby's shoulders fail to deliver shortly after the birth of the baby's head, and is treated by supra-pubic pressure, change of maternal position, or internal turning of the baby to release its posterior shoulder.

Systematic review: a structured literature review that collects and critically analyses multiple research studies/papers to answer research questions. A review of existing studies is often quicker and cheaper than embarking on a new study and systematic reviews are an important element of health care research.

Type 1 diabetes: a form of diabetes that results from auto-immune destruction of the beta-cells in the pancreas that produce insulin. The resulting lack of insulin leads to increased glucose in blood and urine and symptoms of frequent urination, increased thirst and hunger and weight loss. The cause of type 1 diabetes is unknown. Administration of insulin is essential for survival and must be continued indefinitely. People with type 1 diabetes usually manage their diabetes independently. Poorly treated diabetes can cause many complications including diabetic ketoacidosis and coma. Serious long-term complications related to hyperglycaemia include heart disease, stroke, renal failure, foot ulcers and damage to the eyes. Type 1 diabetes accounts for between 5% and 10% of all diabetes cases. Globally, about 80,000 children develop the disease each year but it can also occur in adulthood.

Type 2 diabetes: a metabolic disorder characterised by hyperglycaemia, insulin resistance, and a relative lack of insulin. Symptoms may come on more slowly but longer-term complications are similar to those of type 1 diabetes above. Type 2 diabetes is primarily due to increased BMI and not enough exercise in people who are genetically predisposed, so is partly preventable by weight loss, a healthy diet and regular exercise. Type 2 diabetes makes up about 90% of cases of diabetes. Treatment involves lifestyle changes and, if these do not lower blood glucose levels adequately, metformin. Many people may eventually also require insulin injections.

WHO/World Health Organisation: the agency of the United Nations concerned with international public health, established in 1948 and headquartered in Geneva, Switzerland.

References

Agro M & Fillmore H (2014). Screening for Hyperglycemia in Pregnancy: Standardizing the Breakfast challenge. *Midwifery Matters*, 1 (1) 4-10, Summer 2014.

Allen R, Schwartzman E, Baker W, Coleman C, Phung O (2013). Cinnamon use in type 2 diabetes: an updated systematic review and meta-analysis.' *Annals of Family Medicine*, 11 (5), 452-9, Sept/Oct 2013. doi:10.1370/afm.1517.

Alwan N, Tuffnell D, West J (2009). Treatments for gestational diabetes. *Cochrane Database Systematic Review*, July 2009. doi:10.1002/14651858. CD003395.pub2.

Aroda V, Christophi C, Edelstein S, Zhang P, Herman W, Barrett-Connor E, Delahanty L, Montez M, Ackermann R, Zhuo X, Knowler W, Ratner R (2015). The Effect of Lifestyle Intervention and Metformin on Preventing or Delaying Diabetes Among Women With and Without Gestational Diabetes: The Diabetes Prevention Program Outcomes Study 10-Year Follow-Up. *The Journal of Clinical Endocrinology and Metabolism,* February 23, 2015 *http://press. endocrine.org/doi/abs/10.1210/jc.2014-3761*

Balsells M, Garcia-Patterson A, Solà I, Roqué M, Gich I, Corcoy R (2015). 'Glibenclamide, metformin, and insulin for the treatment of gestational diabetes: a systematic review and meta-analysis.' *British Medical Journal*, 350, h102, 1-12, January 2015. doi: 10.1136/bmj.h102

Bertoldo M, Faure M, Dupont J, Froment P (2014). Impact of metformin on reproductive tissues: an overview from gametogenesis to gestation.' *Annals of Translational Medicine, 2* (6) June 2014 doi: 10.3978/j.issn.2305-5839.2014.06.04

Beyerlein A, Schiessl B, Lack N et al. Associations of gestational weight loss with birth-related outcome: a retrospective cohort study. *BJOG,* 2011, 118, 55–61.

Buchanan T, Xiang A, Peters R. et al. (2002). Preservation of pancreatic ß cell function and prevention of type 2 diabetes by pharmacological treatment of insulin resistance in high-risk Hispanic women. *Diabetes,* 51, 2796–2803.

Chang S, Lin K, Lin R, Hung P, Lin J, Cheng J (2006). Enhanced insulin sensitivity using electroacupuncture on bilateral Zusanli acupoints (ST36) in rats.' *Life Sciences,* 70 (10), 967-71, August 2006.

Chiswick C and 14 others (2015). Effect of metformin on maternal and fetal outcomes in obese pregnant women (EMPOWaR): a randomised, duble-blind, placebo-controlled trial. *The Lancet Diabetes & Endocrinology*, 3 (10), 778-786, October 2015.

Chu S, Callaghan W, Kim S *et al.* (2007). Maternal obesity and risk of gestational diabetes mellitus, *Diabetes Care*, 30 (8) 2070–2076.

Cochrane Pregnancy and Childbirth (2016). Induction of labour for big babies. Infographic by Helen West, available from http://pregnancy.cochrane.org/sites/pregnancy.cochrane.org/files/uploads/induction-for-macrosomia%20(screen).pdf

Corcoy R, personal communication, December 2015.

De-Regil M, Palacios C, Lombardo L, Pena-Rosas J. (2016).'Vitamin D supplementation for women during pregnancy.' Cochrane Pregnancy & Childbirth Group. 14.1.16. DOI:10.1002/14651858.CD008873.pub3iabetes UK (2011) Evidence-based Nutrition

Donazar-Ezcurra M, Lopez-Burgo C, Bes-Rastrollo M (2017). Primary prevention of gestational diabetes mellitus through nutritional factors: a systematic review. *BMC Pregnancy and Childbirth*, 17 (30), 13.1.17. DOI:10.1186/s12884-016-1205-4

Dornhorst A, Paterson C, Nicholls J, Wadsworth J, Chiu D, Elkeles R, *et al.* (1992). High Prevalence of Gestational Diabetes in Women from Ethnic Minority Groups. *Diabetic Medicine,* 9, 820–5.

Farrar D, Fairley L, Santorelli G, Tuffnell D, Sheldon T, Wright J, van Overveld L, Lawlor D (2015). Association between hyperglycaemia and adverse perinatal outcomes in south Asian and white British women: analysis of data from the Born in Bradford cohort. *Lancet Diabetes & Endocrinology,* 3 (10), 795-804, October 2015.

Feig D (2012). Drugs and breastfeeding in women with diabetes, in Lindsay R (ed.) *Diabetes in Pregnancy.* Oxford University Press.

Gilinsky A, Kirk A, Hughes A and Lindsay R (2015). Lifestyle interventions for type 2 diabetes prevention in women with prior gestational diabetes: A systematic review and meta-analysis of behavioural, anthropometric and metabolic outcomes. *Preventive Medicine Reports* 2, 2015, 448-461.

Gunderson E, Hurston S, Ning X, Lo J, Crites Y, Walton D, Dewey K, Azevedo R, Young S, Fox G, Elmasian C, Salvador N, Lum M, Sternfeld B, Quesenberry C (2015). Lactation and Progression to Type 2 Diabetes Mellitus After

Gestational Diabetes Mellitus. A Prospective Cohort Study. *Annals of Internal Medicine*, 163 (12):1-36. doi:10.7326/P15-9038.

The HAPO Study Cooperative Research Group (2008). Hyperglycemia and Adverse Pregnancy Outcomes. *New England Journal of Medicine*, 358:1991-2002, May 2008. DOI: 10.1056/NEJMoa0707943.

Hernandez T, Friedman J, Van Pelt R, Barbour L (2011). Patterns of Glycaemia in Normal Pregnancy. *Diabetes Care*, 34, 1660-1668, July 2011.

IADPSG Consensus Panel (2010). International Association of Diabetes and Pregnancy Study Groups Recommendations on the Diagnosis and Classification of Hyperglycaemia in Pregnancy. *Diabetes Care*, 33 (3), 676-682, March 2010.

Ignell C, Ekelund M, Anderberg E, Berntorp K (2016). Model for individual prediction of diabetes up to 5 years after gestational diabetes mellitus. *Springer Plus*, 5: 318. doi:10.1186/s40064-016-1953-7.

InFact (2006). Risks of Formula Feeding. (http://www.infactcanada.ca/ RisksofFormulaFeeding.pdf)

Kim C (2014). Maternal outcomes and follow-up after gestational diabetes mellitus. *Diabetic Medicine*, 31 (3), 292-301, March 2014. doi: 10.1111/ dme.12382

Landon, M, Spong C, Thom E, Carpenter M, Ramin S, Casey B, Wapner R, Varner M, Rouse D, Thorp J, Sciscione A, Catalano P, Harper M, Saade G, Lain K, Sorokin Y, Peaceman A, Tolosa J, Anderson G. (2009) A Multicenter, Randomized Trial of Treatment for Mild Gestational Diabetes. *N Engl J Med*, 361:1339-1348, October 2009. DOI: 10.1056/NEJMoa0902430

Lawrence Beech B, Robinson J (1994). *Ultrasound? Unsound.* Association for Improvements in the Maternity Services (available as a .pdf file).

Lawrence Beech B (2003). *Am I Allowed?* Association for Improvements in the Maternity Services.

Lee A *et al.* (2007). Gestational diabetes mellitus: Clinical predictors and long-term risk of developing type 2 diabetes: a retrospective cohort study using survival analysis. *Diabetes Care,* 30.4 (2007): 878-883.

Lindsay R (ed.) (2012). *Diabetes in Pregnancy.* Oxford University Press.

Lindstrom J et al., on behalf of the Finnish Diabetes prevention Study Group (2006). Sustained reduction in the incidence of type 2 diabetes by lifestyle intervention: follow-up of the Finnish Diabetes Prevention Study. *Lancet,* 368 (9548) 1673-79, 11-17

MacKenzie A, Stephenson C, Funai E (2016). Prenatal sonographic assessment of fetal weight. www.uptodate.com/contents/prenatal-sonographic-assessment-of-fetal-weight, updated 4.3.16.

Maghbooli Z, Hossein-Nezhad A, Karimi F, Shafaei A, Larijani B (2007). Correlation between vitamin D3 deficiency and insulin resistance in pregnancy Diabetes/Metabolism *Research and Reviews,* 24 (1) 27-32, 2 July 2007, doi: 10.1002/dmrr.737

Mazze R (2006). *Epidemiology of Diabetes in Pregnancy in The Diabetes in Pregnancy Dilemma: Leading Change with Proven Solutions (ed. Langer O).* University Press of America.

Meek C, Lewis H, Patient C, Murphy H, Simmons D (2015). Diagnosis of gestational diabetes mellitus: falling through the net. *Diabetologia,* doi: 10.1007/s00125-015-3647-z

Metzger BE, Lowe LP, Dyer AR, Trimble ER, Chaovarindr U, Coustan DR *et al.* (2008). Hyperglycemia and adverse pregnancy outcomes. *New England Journal of Medicine,* 358 (19):1991-2002.

Moore E, Anderson G, Bergman N, Dowswell T. (2012). Early skin-to-skin contact for mothers and their healthy newborn infants. *Cochrane Database of Systematic Reviews,* 2012, Issue 5. Art. No.: CD003519. DOI: 10.1002/14651858. CD003519.pub3.

Morton S, Kirkwood S, Thangaratinam S. (2014). Interventions to modify the progression to type 2 diabtes mellitus in women with gestational diabetes: a systematic review of literature. *Current Opinion in Obstetrics and Gynecology,* 26, 476-486 December 2014.

Moses RG, Calvert D. (1995). Pregnancy outcomes in women without gestational diabetes mellitus related to the maternal glucose level. Is there a continuum of risk? *Diabetes Care,* 18(12):1527-1533.

Much D, Beyerlein A and 15 others (2016). Lactation is associated with altered metabolomic signatures in women with gestational diabetes. *Diabetologica,* pp 1-10, published online 16.7.2016. doi: 10.1007/s00125-016-4055-8.

NICE (2008). 'Inducing labour. NICE guidelines' [CG70] July 2008

NICE (2015). 'Diabetes in Pregnancy: management of diabetes and its complications from preconception to the postnatal period' [NG3] February 2015

NIHR (National Institute for Health Research) (2016). 'On the level: Evidence for action on type 2 diabetes.' NIHR Dissemination Centre, September 2016.

Poston L, Bell R, Croker H, Flynn A, Godfrey K, Goff L, Hayes L, Khazaezadeh N, Nelson S, Oteng-Ntim E, Pasupathy D, Patel N, Robson S, Sandall J, Sanders T, Sattar N, Seed P, Wardle J, Whitworth M, Briley A & UPBEAT Trial Consortium (2015). Effect of a behavioural intervention in obese pregnant women (the UPBEAT study): a multicentre, randomised controlled trial. *The Lancet Diabetes and Endocrinology*, 3 (10), 767-777. doi: 10.1016/S2213-8587(15)00227-2.

Poston L (2016). The UPBEAT trial: behavioural intervention in obese pregnant women. Presentation at the 5th National Diabetes in Pregnancy Conference, London 10.11.16.

Ratner R. (2006). An update on the Diabetes Prevention Program. *Endocrine Practice*, 12 (Supplement 1), 20-24. doi: 10.4158/EP.12S1.20

Ratner RE, Christophi CA, Metzger BE, Dabelea D, Bennett PH, *et al.* (2008). Prevention of diabetes in women with a history of gestational diabetes: effects of metformin and lifestyle interventions. *J Clin Endocrinol Metab*, 93, 4774–4779.

Rayanagoudar G, Hashi A, Zamora J, Khan K, Hitman G, Thangaratinam S (2016). Quantification of the type 2 diabetes risk in women with gestational diabetes: a systematic review and meta-analysis of 95,750 women. *Diabetologica* 59, 1403-11, April 2016. doi:10.1007/s00125-016-3927-2.

Rogozinska E, Chamillard M, Hitman G, Khan K, Thangaratinam S (2015). Nutritional Manipulation for the Primary Prevention of Gestational Diabetes Mellitus: A Meta-Analysis of Randomised Studies. PLoS ONE 10 (2) e0115526. doi:10.1371/journal.pone.0115526

Rosenstein M, Cheng Y, Snowden J, Nicholson J, Doss A, Caughey A (2012). The risk of Stillbirth and Infant Death Stratified by Gestational Age in Women with Gestational Diabetes. *Am J Obstet Gynecol*. April 2012, 206 (4) 309. doi:10.1016/j.ajog.2012.01.014

Rowan J, Hague W, Gao W, Battin M, Moore M (2008). Metformin versus insulin for the treatment of gestational diabetes. *New England Journal of Medicine*, 358, 2003-15.

Rowan J, Rush E, Obolonkin V, Battin M, Wouldes T, Hague W. (2011). Metformin in Gestational Diabetes: The Offspring Follow-Up (MiG TOFU). *Diabetes Care*, 34 (10), 2279-2284, October 2011. doi:10.2337/dc11-0660.

RCOG (2013). Shoulder Dystocia, March 2013 *www.rcog.org.uk/globalassets/ documents/patients/patient-information-leaflets/pregnancy/pi-shoulder-dystocia.pdf*

Sanabria-Martínez G, *et al.* (2015). Effectiveness of physical activity interventions on preventing gestational diabetes mellitus and excessive maternal weight gain: a meta-analysis. *BJOG*, 2015;122:1167–1174

Sanghi, A (2016). 'Designing community-based pathways for GDM care.' Presentation at The 5th National Diabetes in Pregnancy Conference, London 10.11.16.

Siega-Riz AM, Viswanathan M, Moos MK *et al.* (2009). A systematic review of outcomes of maternal weight gain according to the Institute of Medicine's recommendations: birthweight, fetal growth, and postpartum weight retention. *American Journal of Obstetrics and Gynecology*, 201: 339 e1–14

Simmons D (2010). Diabetes and obesity in pregnancy. *Best Practice and Research Clinical Obstetrics and Gynaecology*. 25.10.2010 doi:10.1016/j. bpopgyn.2010.10.006

Simmons D, and 23 others (2016). Effect of physical activity and/or healthy eating on GDM risk: The DALI Lifestyle Study. *The Journal of Clinical Endocrinology & Metabolism*, December 2016.

Song C, Li J, Leng J, Ma R, Yang X (2016). Lifestyle intervention can reduce the risk of gestational diabetes: a meta-analysis of randomised controlled trials. *World Obesity*, 17, 960-969, October 2016. doi:10.111/0br.12442.

Sovio U, Murphy H, Smith G (2016). Accelerated Fetal Growth Prior to Diagnosis of Gestational Diabetes Mellitus: A Prospective Cohort Study of Nulliparous Women. *Diabetes Care*, 39 (6), 982-7, June 2016.

Stewart Z (2014) Gestational Diabetes. Medical Observer Talking Women, 26.9.14, 27-28. *www.jeanhailes.org.au*

Syngelaki A, Nicolaides K, Balani J, Hyer S, Akolekar R, Kotecha R, Pastides A, Shehata H (2016). Metformin versus Placebo in Obese Pregnant Women without Diabetes Mellitus. *New England Journal of Medicine*, 374:434-443, 4.2.16. DOI: 10.1056/NEJMoa1509819

Unwin D & Unwin J (2014). Low carbohydrate diet to achieve weight loss and improve HbA1c in type 2 diabetes and pre-diabetes: experience from one general practice. *Practical Diabetes*, 31 (2), 76-79, March 2014. doi:10.1002/pdi.1835.

Wickham S (2014). *Inducing Labour: Making Informed Decisions*. Association for Improvements in the Maternity Services.

World Health Organisation (2013). 'Diagnostic Criteria and Classification of Hyperglycaemia First Detected in Pregnancy' WHO/NMH/MND/13.2

Zeigler A, Wallner M, Kaiser I, Rossbauer M, Harsunen M, Lachmann L, Maier J, Winkler C, Hummel S. (2012). Long-Term Protective Effect of Lactation on the Development of Type 2 Diabetes in Women With Recent Gestational Diabetes Mellitus. *Diabetes*, 2012;61:3167–3171.

About the Author

Deborah Hughes

Deborah Hughes has worked mainly as a community-based and independent midwife since 1982, and has been a member of AIMS for nearly as long. Her midwifery interests focus on physiological pregnancy and birth, attachment parenting, and issues of self-determination, autonomy and choice for women, and support for midwives. She currently works as a research midwife in Cambridge. Deborah has had many articles published in a variety of midwifery journals and one previous book: *Tensions and Barriers in Improving Maternity Care* (co-authored with Ruth Deery and Mavis Kirkham) which explored the factors leading to birth centre closure.

About the Illustrator

Jennifer Williams

Jennifer Williams is an American artist based in London. She is a member of the International Futures Forum (IFF). As a lifelong maker, her artwork ranges from handmade books, cutouts, photographs, illustration and printmaking to the making of puppets and masks. She has illustrated books for authors throughout the UK, USA and India including *Equal Exposure* (Glasgow Centre for Population Health) *Many Futures of India* (Academic Foundation, Delhi), *Economies of Life*, *Dancing at the Edge*, *Three Horizons*, *Humanising Healthcare* and *Transformational Innovation* (IFF/Triarchy Press).

Other publications published by AIMS can be ordered from our website – www.aims.org.uk/?pubs.htm

Please let us know your views of this book by emailing: feedback@aims.org.uk

- *Am I Allowed?*
- *Birth After Caesarean*
- *Birthing Your Baby: The Second Stage*
- *Birthing Your Placenta: The Third Stage*
- *Breech Birth - What are my options?*
- *Inducing Labour - Making Informed Decisions*
- *Group B Strep Explained*
- *Safety in Childbirth*
- *Making a Complaint about Maternity Care*
- *Vitamin K and the Newborn*
- *Caesarean Birth - Your Questions Answered*

We are pleased to offer some of these books as Kindle files which are available from Amazon.

AiMS

There for your mother

Here for you

Help us to be there for your daughters

www.aims.org.uk

Twitter – @AIMS_online

Facebook – www.facebook.com/AIMSUK

Helpline

helpline@aims.org.uk

0300 365 0663

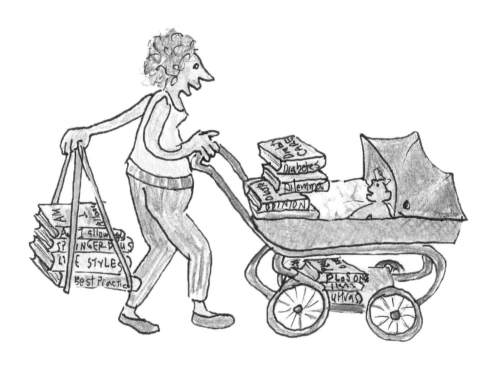